Voluntary Termination of Pregnancy

Advances in Reproductive Health Care

(1984/85)

E. S. E. Hafez: Series Editor

LHRH and Its Analogs: Contraception and Therapeutic Applications
H. Vickery, J. J. Nestor, Jr. and E. S. E. Hafez (editors)

Spontaneous Abortion
E. S. E. Hafez (editor)

Voluntary Termination of Pregnancy
E. S. E. Hafez (editor)

Biomedical Aspects of IUDs
H. Hasson, W. A. A. van Os and E. S. E. Hafez (editors)

Prostaglandins and Fertility Regulation
M. Toppozada, M. Bygdeman and E. S. E. Hafez (editors)

Male Fertility and Its Regulation
T. Lobl and E. S. E. Hafez (editors)

Advances in
Reproductive Health Care

Voluntary Termination of Pregnancy

Editor

E. S. E. Hafez

Reproductive Health Center and
IVF/Andrology International

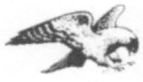 **MTP PRESS LIMITED**
a member of the KLUWER ACADEMIC PUBLISHERS GROUP
LANCASTER / BOSTON / THE HAGUE / DORDRECHT

Published in the UK and Europe by
MTP Press Limited
Falcon House
Lancaster, England

British Library Cataloguing in Publication Data

Voluntary termination of pregnancy.—
  (Advances in reproductive health care;
  1. Abortion
  I. Hafez, E. S. E.   II. Series
  618.8'8   RG734

Published in the USA by
MTP Press
A division of Kluwer Boston Inc
190 Old Derby Street
Hingham, MA 02043, USA

Library of Congress Cataloging in Publication Data

Main entry under title:

Voluntary termination of pregnancy.

  (Advances in reproductive health care)
  Bibliography: p.
  Includes index.
  1. Abortion.   I. Hafez, E. S. E., 1922–
  II. Series. (DNLM: 1. Abortion, Induced—Congresses.
  WQ 440 V943 1982)
  RG734.V64   1984   618.8'8   84-9691
ISBN-13: 978-94-011-6680-5   e-ISBN-13: 978-94-011-6678-2
DOI: 10.1007/978-94-011-6678-2

Contents

List of Contributors

H. ABRAMOVICI
Department of Obstetrics and Gynecology,
Carmel Medical Center,
Haifa 34362, Israel

M. M. AHMAD
Department of Obstetrics and Gynecology,
The University of Texas Health Science
    Center at San Antonio,
7703 Floyd Curl Drive, San Antonio,
Texas 78284, USA

A. M. ALTMAN
Department of Obstetrics and Gynecology,
Harvard Medical School and Brigham and
    Women's Hospital (formerly the Boston
    Hospital for Women),
Boston, Massachusetts, USA

J. T. ANDERSEN
Department of Gynecology and Obstetrics,
Gentofte and Herlev Hospitals,
University of Copenhagen, Denmark

J. ATAD
Department of Obstetrics and Gynecology,
Carmel Medical Center,
Haifa 34362, Israel

M. M. BAYLSON
Duane, Morris and Heckscher,
One Franklin Plaza,
Philadelphia 19102, USA

J. BONTIS
First Department of Obstetrics and
    Gynecology,
Aristotelian University of Thessaloniki
    Medical School,
Thessaloniki, Greece

R. C. BRIEL
Department of Obstetrics and Gynecology,

University of Tuebingen,
D-7400 Tuebingen, FRG

V. J. CZIGREIENE
Department of Obstetrics and Gynecology,
Kaunas Medical Institute,
Kaunas-233007 Eivieniu 2,
Lithuanian SSR, USSR

E. M. DERKS-HAMMELBURG
Elisabeth Gasthius, Boerhaavelaan 22,
Haarlem, The Netherlands

M. P. EMBREY
Nuffield Department of
    Obstetrics/Gynaecology,
John Radcliffe Hospital,
Headington,
Oxford OX3 9DU, UK

J. H. FAKTOR
Department of Obstetrics and Gynecology,
Carmel Medical Center,
Haifa 34362, Israel

M. FILICORI
Vincent Research Laboratories,
Department of Gynecology,
Massachusetts General Hospital,
Boston, Massachusetts 02114, USA

C. FLAMIGNI
Department of Reproductive Medicine,
University of Bologna,
Via Massarenti 13,
40138 Bologna, Italy

S. P. GOLDSTEIN
Department of Obstetrics and Gynecology,
Harvard Medical School and the Brigham
    and Women's Hospital (formerly the
    Boston Hospital for Women),
Boston, Massachusetts, USA

LIST OF CONTRIBUTORS

E. S. E. HAFEZ
IVF/Andrology International,
Reproductive Health Center
Medical University of
South Carolina,
171 Ashley, Charleston,
SC 29425, USA

R. HALLIWELL
MRC Medical Sociology Unit,
Institute of Medical Sociology,
Westburn Road, Aberdeen AB9 2ZE,
Scotland, UK

L. HEISTERBERG
Departments of Gynecology and
Obstetrics,
Gentofte and Herlev Hospitals,
University of Copenhagen, Denmark

R. ILLSLEY
MRC Medical Sociology Unit,
Institute of Medical Sociology,
Westburn Road, Aberdeen AB9 2ZE,
Scotland, UK

C. A. INGEMANSON
Obstetrics and Gynecology Department,
Central Hospital, Eskilstuna,
Sweden

N. KLEARCHOU
First Department of Obstetrics and
Gynecology,
Aristotelian University of Thessaloniki
Medical School,
Thessaloniki, Greece

W. KUHN
Department of Gynecology and Obstetrics,
University Göttingen, Humboldtalle 3,
D-3400 Göttingen, FRG

H. KÜHNLE
Department of Gynecology and Obstetrics,
University Göttingen, Humboldtalle 3,
D-3400 Göttingen, FRG

I. Z. MACKENZIE
Nuffield Department of
Obstetrics/Gynaecology,
John Radcliffe Hospital, Headington,
Oxford OX3 9DU, UK

Y. MANABE
Department of Obstetrics and Gynecology,
Kyoto University School of Medicine,
Sakyo-Ku, Kyoto 606, Japan

S. MANTALENAKIS
First Department of Obstetrics and
Gynecology,
Aristotelian University of Thessaloniki
Medical School,
Thessaloniki, Greece

A. NAKAJIMA
Department of Obstetrics and Gynecology,
Ehime University School of Medicine,
Ehime 791, Japan

H. NISHIMURA
Central Institute for Experimental Animals,
Miyamae-Ku, Kawasaki 213, Japan

W. RATH
Department of Gynecology and Obstetrics,
University Göttingen, Humboldtalle 3,
D-3400 Göttingen, FRG

P. E. R. RHEMREV
Department of Gynecology and Obstetrics,
Elisabeth Gasthius, Boerhaavelaan 22,
Haarlem, The Netherlands

A. ROFE
Department of Obstetrics and Gynecology,
Carmel Medical Center,
Haifa 34362, Israel

V. M. SADAUSKAS
Department of Obstetrics and Gynecology,
Kaunas Medical Institute,
Kaunas-233007 Eivieniu 2,
Lithuanian SSR, USSR

E. SAVIOTTI
Department of Reproductive Medicine,
University of Bologna, Via Massarenti 13,
40138 Bologna, Italy

K. SHIOTA
Congenital Anomaly Research Center,
Faculty of Medicine, Kyoto University,
Kyoto 606, Japan

S. SONNE-HOLM
Department of Gynecology and Obstetrics,
Gentofte and Herlev Hospitals,
University of Copenhagen, Denmark

P. G. STUBBLEFIELD
Department of Obstetrics and Gynecology,
Harvard Medical School and the Brigham
and Women's Hospital (formerly Boston
Hospital for Women),
Boston, Massachusetts, USA

LIST OF CONTRIBUTORS

B. THOMPSON
MRC Medical Sociology Unit,
Institute of Medical Sociology,
Westburn Road, Aberdeen AB9 2ZE,
Scotland, UK

W. A. A. VAN OS
Department of Gynecology and Obstetrics,
Elisabeth Gasthuis, Boerhaavelaan 22,
Haarlem, The Netherlands

Y. YOSHIDA
Department of Obstetrics and Gynecology,
Shiga University of Medical School,
Shiga 520, Japan

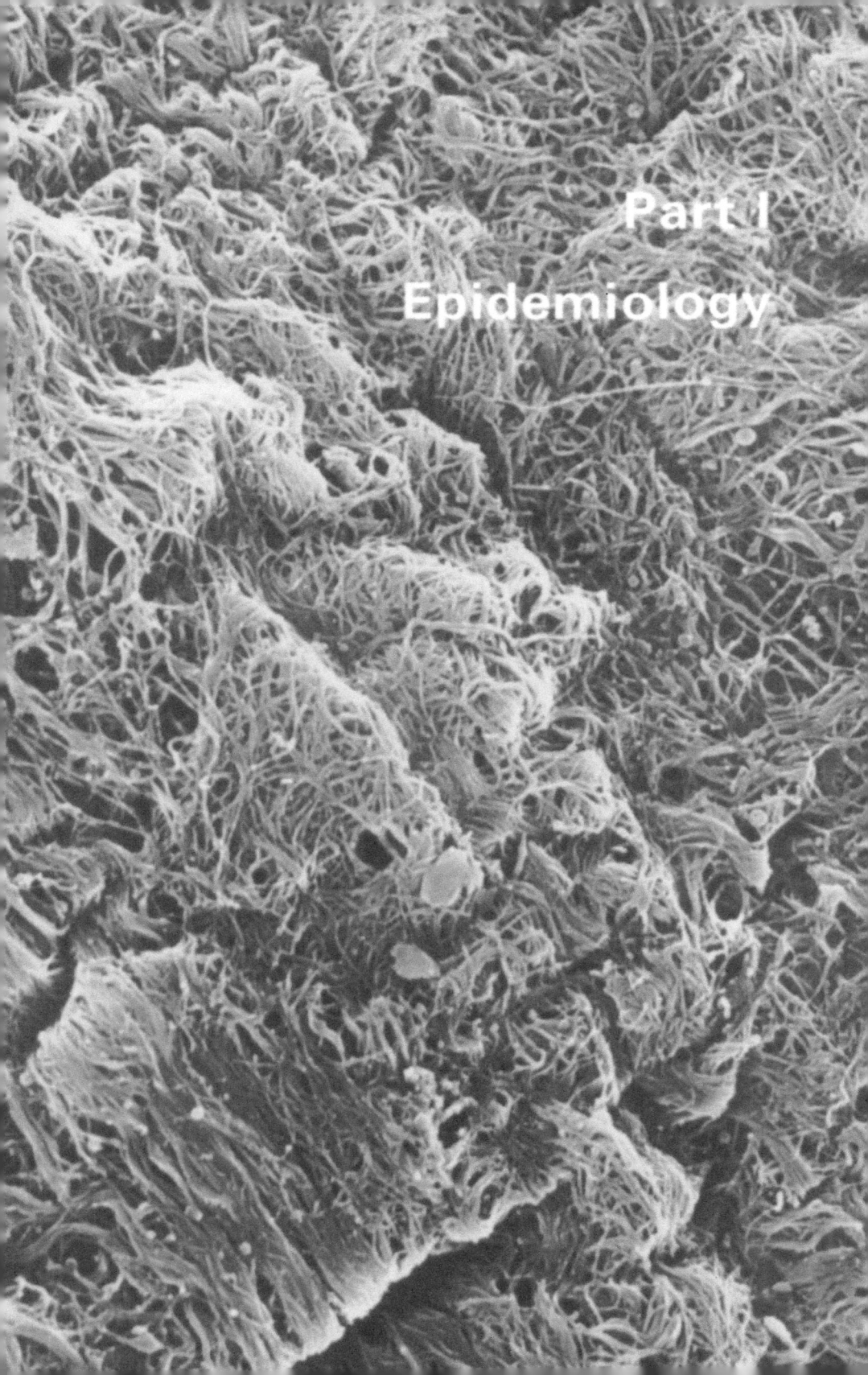

Part I

Epidemiology

1

Epidemiology of induced abortion in Japan

K. SHIOTA and H. NISHIMURA

Japan is one of the countries having a long history of legal abortion. Artificial interruption of pregnancies has been legally permitted in Japan since 1948 when the Eugenic Protection Law was passed by the Diet. The law was adopted to make it possible to perform abortions under sanitary, safe conditions instead of illegal abortions performed under very bad conditions. It was also aimed at the prevention of overpopulation and the birth of undesirable offspring from the eugenic viewpoint. In 1949 an important amendment was made, whereby economic factors were added to the legal basis of abortion. Article 14 of the law reads in part:

> The physician designated by the Medical Association . . . may perform an artificial termination of pregnancy on anyone coming under any of the following items with the consent of the person in question and the spouse: . . . Paragraph 4. If the health of the mother may be seriously affected by the continuation of pregnancy or the delivery due to her physical or economic condition.

Under the legalization, roughly 1 million abortions on the average have been reported annually.

There have been several studies on the demographic aspects of induced abortion in Japan. Although most of them were based on data from the Eugenic Protection Statistics, the completeness of reporting from physicians on which the statistics depend has been subject to serious suspicions. Thus, in this chapter, two sets of data were employed for analysis of the Japanese data: (1) The Eugenic Protection Statistics (EPS), which are official statistics published annually by the Ministry of Health and Welfare of Japan. The only maternal data available in the statistics are age and gestational week at abortion. (2) The data regarding approximately 7000 human embryos procured mainly for 'socioeconomic' reasons. Nishimura initiated the collection of human conceptuses in 1961, and the collection now comprises nearly 40 000 cases. The details of the collection have been described (Nishimura, 1974, 1975). The specimens have been collected from the broad area of central

Japan, and our embryonic population can be assumed to represent the total population of induced abortuses in Japan. The data presented here are based on a non-selected sample comprising approximately 7000 induced abortuses. Cases with a maternal sign of threatened abortion were excluded, as were hysterotomy/hysterectomy cases. For each specimen, information regarding reproductive and medical histories of the woman was provided by the physician. In the majority of the cases pregnancy was terminated by dilatation and curettage in private hospitals or clinics.

In the latter part of the chapter the Japanese data will be compared with corresponding data from the United States which are based on abortion surveys conducted by Alan Guttmacher Institute and the Centers for Disease Control (Henshaw *et al.*, 1981; Tyler, 1981).

DEMOGRAPHIC PATTERNS OF ABORTION IN JAPAN

In 1980 the total number of reported induced abortions in Japan was 598 084 and the rate was 19.6 per 1000 women aged 15−49. Both the total number and the rate of induced abortions have been declining steadily since 1955 (Fig. 1.1).

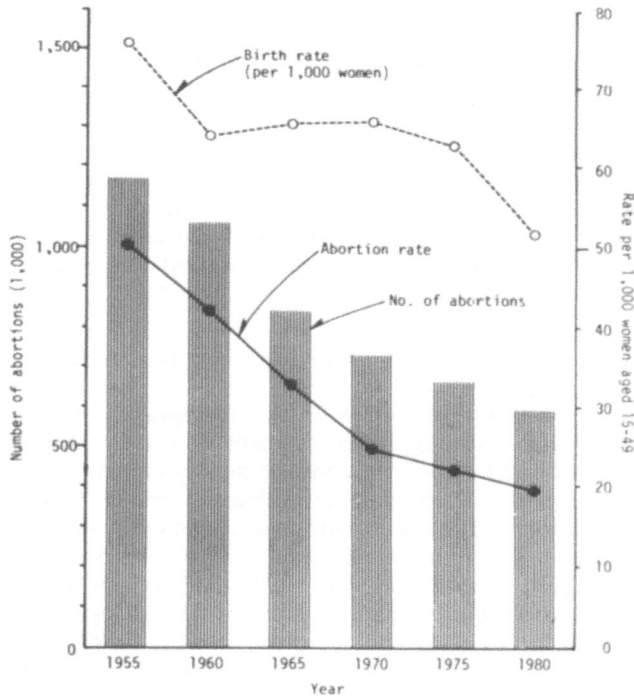

Fig. 1.1 Reported number and rate of induced abortions in Japan (Eugenic Protection Statistics)

The number in 1980 was about half as many as that in 1955. The reporting of induced abortion in Japan is considered inaccurate because physicians may not file all the reports, which could reveal their taxable income, and because patients do not always want to appear on a report. The information as to the induced abortions performed on premarital pregnancies especially is considered far less reliable. The multiplication of the reported number by a factor between 1.5 and 1.7 might give a rough estimation of the total number of abortions actually performed (Muramatsu, 1969). Nevertheless, the decrease in reported induced abortions is believed to represent the true decline rather than a statistical artifact.

The birth rate has also been declining in Japan, mainly due to the recent changes in social circumstances. The average number of children born to a married couple is smaller than 2.0 in recent years. It is possible that induced abortion used to contribute to the fast drop in the birth rate, but its contribution seems to become smaller because the abortion rate has dropped faster than the birth rate. Such a downward trend, both in the abortion and birth rates, was made possible by women's improved knowledge of contraception, and the better accessibility of various contraceptive measures.

The average age of women undergoing abortion is 30.2, which is 2.6 years higher than the average (27.6) for the mothers of all newborns in Japan (Table 1.1). The average age of the mothers of newborns has remained unchanged, with a slight increase noted recently. The average age of the abortion group has declined during recent years. The proportion of women younger than 25 has been increasing. According to the official statistics, the abortion rate has been increasing only in teenagers from 3.1 per thousand women in 1975 to 4.8 in 1980 (Fig. 1.2).

When our embryo data are compared with the Eugenic Protection Statistics, a significant difference is noted in the distributions by maternal age (Fig. 1.3). The proportion of younger women is relatively larger in our embryo collection than in the EPS data. One of the possible explanations for such a difference is that we collected embryos mainly in and around big cities, where people may be less conservative than in rural areas. This, however, does not solely explain the difference because cultural circumstances inside Japan

Table 1.1 Percentage distribution of induced abortions in Japan, by maternal age[1]

| Year | Maternal age (in years) | | | | | | | Total | Mean age | Mean for total livebirths[2] |
	<20	20–24	25–29	30–34	35–39	40–44	>44			
1961–65	1.6	20.1	27.5	27.4	16.2	6.9	0.3	100.0	30.4	27.5
1966–70	2.4	20.4	27.9	26.2	17.5	5.2	0.4	100.0	30.2	27.5
1971–75	2.8	23.6	22.7	25.1	18.4	7.1	0.3	100.0	30.2	27.5
1976–80	5.6	22.5	23.6	22.1	18.6	6.7	0.9	100.0	30.0	27.9
Total	3.0	21.7	25.4	25.3	17.8	6.3	0.5	100.0	30.2[3] ± 6.2 (SD)	27.6 ± 4.5 (SD)

[1] Human embryo data
[2] Vital statistics data
[3] Significantly different from livebirths ($p < 0.01$)

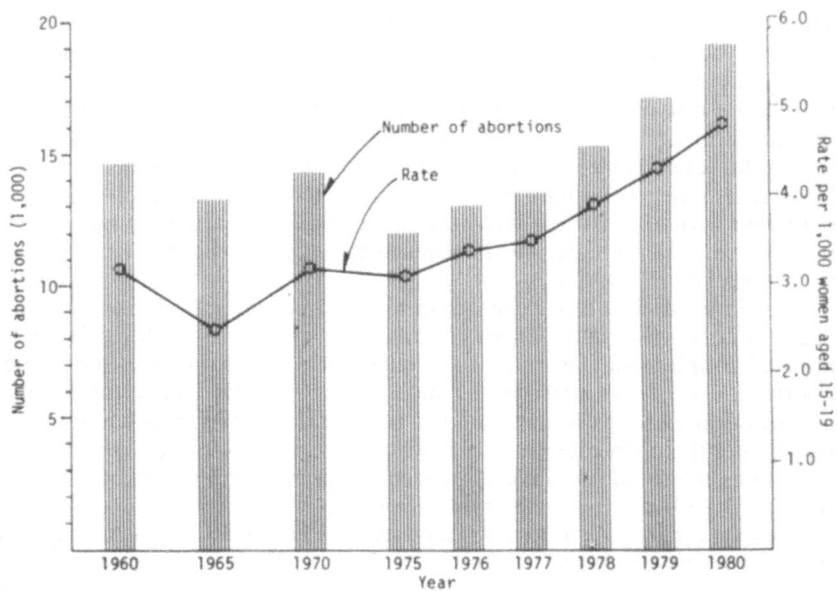

Fig. 1.2 Reported number and rate of induced abortions in teenage women in Japan (Eugenic Protection Statistics)

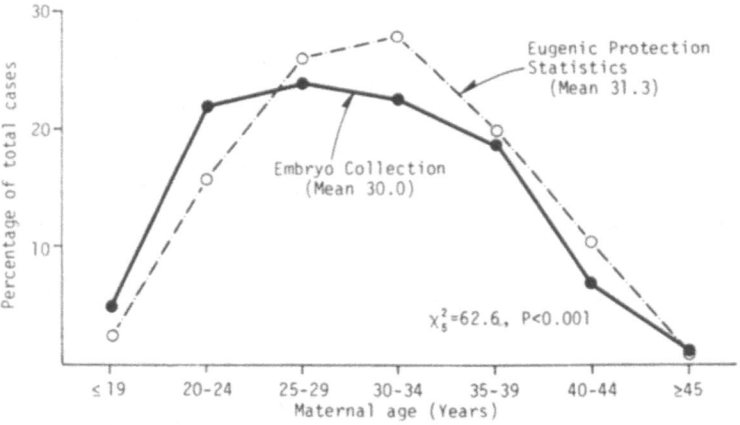

Fig. 1.3 Distribution of induced abortions in Japan by maternal age, 1976–1980

are considered quite uniform these days. An alternative explanation which seems more probable is that the rate of reporting (or under-reporting) might be different by women's age groups. Abortions obtained by unmarried young women might be less completely reported due to the difficulty in paperwork. Thus our embryo data would more accurately represent the total population

Table 1.2 Number of living children in women undergoing induced abortion[1]

| Year | Mean no. of children | Number of children | | | |
		0 (%)	1 (%)	≥ 2 (%)	Total (%)
1961–65	1.71	21	23	56	100
1966–70	1.48	26	22	52	100
1971–75	1.48	28	19	53	100
1976–80	1.20[2]	41[2]	15	44	100
Total	1.47[3]	28	20	52[3]	100
Mothers of newborns[4] (1978)	0.77	41	42	17	100

[1] Human embryo data
[2] Significantly different from other groups ($p < 0.05$)
[3] Significantly different from newborns ($p < 0.01$)
[4] Vital statistics data

of induced abortuses in Japan. If this assumption is correct, the proportion of teenagers would actually be larger than officially reported. For example, teenagers account for 5.6 % of the total cases in 1976–80 according to our embryo data instead of 2.5 % from the EPS data for the corresponding period.

More than half of the women undergoing abortion had two or more children, while only 17 % of the mothers of a newborn baby had two or more (Table 1.2). The average number of children of the women in the abortion group has been decreasing, especially during recent years. The proportion of

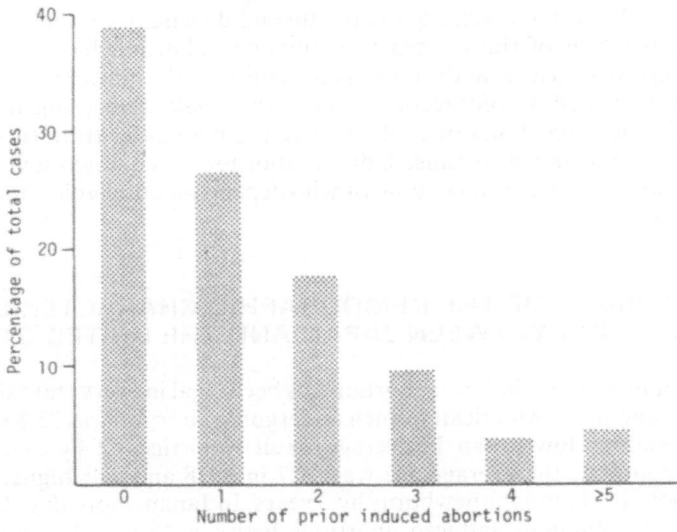

Fig. 1.4 Prior induced abortions in women undergoing abortion in Japan, 1961–1980

the women with no children increased from 21 % in 1961–65 to 41 % in 1976–80. These findings, together with the age data above, mean that in Japan induced abortion has been obtained mainly by married women who already have children, but this characteristic seems to be changing very recently. In other words, the proportion of abortions obtained by young, childless women is becoming larger.

Sixty one per cent of the women who asked for abortion had one or more induced abortions prior to the index case (Fig. 1.4). The average number of previous abortions was 1.3. According to a survey conducted by the health authorities in 1964, four out of ten women aged 20–39 admitted having experienced at least one induced abortion, and the proportion with such experience increased with the women's age and the number of children they have (cited from Muramatsu, 1969).

The proportion of abortions in the first pregnancy showed a significant increase from 11 % in the early 1960s to 26 % in the late 1970s. This trend is obvious especially after 1975. The proportion of primigravid women increased rapidly from 20 % in 1976 to 32 % in 1980. Such rapid changes in the characteristics of the Japanese women undergoing abortion may be attributed to the facts that the abortions obtained by married women are decreasing and that young people are becoming sexually more active.

Over 95 % of the total abortions were performed by the end of the twelfth week of menstrual age. More than two-thirds of the total cases were performed between the seventh and the ninth weeks of gestation. These features have changed little during the last two decades. It should be noted that in Japan induced abortion is seldom provided for menstrual regulation. In Japan, where abortions are performed mostly in the first trimester, abortion-related deaths are reported very rarely and the rate is lower than 1 per 100 000 cases. It is also admitted that Japanese physicians are generally skillful, and that their techniques are safe and dependable (Neubardt, 1977).

Sixty per cent of the women who obtained abortion had employed no contraceptive measures at the time of conception of the index case. Among the women who used a contraception, more than half were using the rhythm method. The percentages of contraceptive use may differ from those for the total women in Japan, because induced abortion is requested mainly by the women who use no contraception, or who depend on unreliable contraceptive measures.

COMPARISON OF THE DEMOGRAPHIC CHARACTERISTICS OF ABORTION BETWEEN JAPAN AND THE UNITED STATES

In the United States, induced abortion has been legal in every state since 1973. The average age of American women undergoing abortion was 23.8 in the year of 1978 and was lower than the average for all livebirths by 2.4 years. In Japan, on the contrary, the average age was 29.7 in 1978 and was higher than the corresponding figure for newborns by 2 years. In Japan, more than half of the women are obtaining induced abortions between 25 and 34 years of age, whereas in the United States nearly two-thirds of the women are younger than

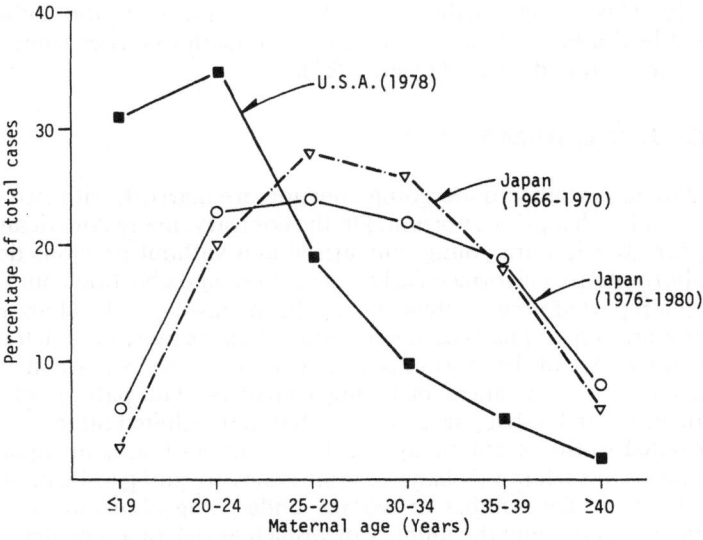

Fig. 1.5 Distributions of induced abortions by maternal age, Japan and the United States

25 (Fig. 1.5). The proportion of teenagers has remained at 3–6 % in Japan, although it is now increasing. It is as high as 31 % in the United States.

With regard to the number of living children, the largest percentage was recorded in women who have no children in the United States (57 % in 1978). In Japan many abortions used to be obtained by women who had two or more children, but recently the proportion of nulliparous women is becoming greater (Table 1.2). The proportion of the women who had at least one induced abortion prior to the index case was 61 % in Japan but only 29 % in the United States.

In Japan more than 95 % of the total abortions were performed by the end of the third month of gestation (Table 1.3). In the United States the proportion of mid-trimester abortions is still larger than in Japan, but is decreasing

Table 1.3 Distribution of induced abortions in Japan and the United States, by gestational stage at termination

Weeks of gestation[1]	Japan (%)		USA (%)	
	1973	1978	1973	1978
≤ 8	59	59	36	52
9–12	38	36	47	39
13–15	1	2	7	4
≥ 16	2	2	10	5
Total	100	100	100	100

[1] Weeks since last menstrual period

gradually. This change in the States should have a favorable influence on maternal health because the abortion-related death rate rises sharply as the stage of gestation advances (Tyler, 1981).

CONCLUDING REMARKS

Many Japanese women undergoing abortion are married, with two or more children and with a prior abortion. On the contrary, many American women asking for abortion are young, unmarried and without previous deliveries. Most abortions are performed early in gestation, and abortion complications have been reported very rarely in Japan. In the history of legal abortion for over 30 years, Japan has experienced rapid changes most of which occurred very recently. One of the most important changes is the increase in abortions obtained by young women, including teenagers. The pattern of induced abortion in Japan has become similar to that in the United States, and it may be attributed to the recent changes in social circumstances in Japan.

As a result of such rapid changes, some issues are going to be important in Japan. First, as the number of women undergoing abortion in their first pregnancy is increasing, the number of women at risk of a repeated abortion also continues to increase. Second, there is a problem of the increasing number of teenagers. Since more teenagers are experiencing induced abortion, the influence of abortion on their premature reproductive system is important. Continued epidemiologic surveillance is needed to assess the possible influences of the changing patterns of abortion on the health of women of childbearing age.

Acknowledgments

We gratefully acknowledge the collaboration of several hundred physicians, and of the members of the Congenital Anomaly Research Center and the Department of Anatomy, Kyoto University Faculty of Medicine. Thanks are also due to Miss Chigako Uwabe and Miss Yuko Taniguchi for technical assistance.

References

Henshaw, S., Forrest, J. D., Sullivan, E. and Tietze, C. (1981). Abortion in the United States, 1978–1979. *Fam. Plan. Perspect.*, **13**, 6–18

Muramatsu, M. (1969). The demographic aspects of abortion in Japan. In *Proceedings of the International Population Conference*, London, 1969. Vol. II, pp. 1166–72. The International Union for the Scientific Study of the Population

Neubardt, S. (1977). Mechanical methods of abortion. A personal observation. In Neubardt, S. and Schulman, H. (eds.) *Techniques of Abortion*. pp. 133–40. (Boston: Little, Brown)

Nishimura, H. (1974). Detection of early developmental anomalies in human abortuses. In Gianantonio, C. A. and Berri, G. G. (eds.) *Pediatria XIV*. pp. 159–70. (Buenos Aires: Editorial Medica Panamericana)

Nishimura, H. (1975). Prenatal versus postnatal malformations based on the Japanese experience on induced abortions in the human being. In Blandau, R. J. (ed.) *Aging Gametes*. pp. 349–68. (Basel: S. Karger)

Tyler, C. W., Jr. (1981). Epidemiology of abortion. *J. Reprod. Med.*, **26**, 459–69.

2
Epidemiology of induced abortion in the Middle East

M. M. AHMAD

ISLAM AND ABORTION

The Islamic nations, which constitute about one-fifth of the world population and extend from Morocco to Indonesia, have high birth rates. In much of the Middle East abortion is either completely illegal or permitted only to prevent the woman's death. Only in Kuwait, Morocco and Tunisia are policies less restrictive.

The Jordanian Mofti, Kalkili, in the International Planned Parenthood Federation meeting, said in his 1964 Fatwa that abortion is allowed before 120 days, i.e. before the various organs are differentiated (Kalkili, 1974). After the fourth month it is forbidden unless the mother's life is endangered. Another Fatwa, given in the Arab Republic of Yemen on 23 Moharram, 1288 Hijjriyya, confirms this ruling (Toppozada *et al.*, 1980). Tunisia is one of the few Islamic countries where it has been posssissible to enact a civil law to support the rights of women given to them by the Holy Koran. In 1965 abortion was legalized on social grounds for women with five or more living children. Then, in November 1973, a liberalized abortion law was enforced which makes abortion available, free of charge, for any married or single woman, on the sole basis of her agreement with a legally practising physician (Bchir and Charfeddine, 1978; Charfeddine, 1980). Egypt, in its new modification of the Civil Law, 'Personal Conditions,' also supports women and children in their family rights and restricts liberal divorce and polygamy, but still leaves the abortion status as it was before: 'Punishable, if not done for certified medical reasons' (Law No. 44 of 1979, Cairo, 1979). The Islamic religion forbids deliberate interference with a pregnancy, with the intention of termination, or killing a living organism.

INDUCED ABORTION IN THE MIDDLE EAST

Frequency of occurrence and trends

Induced abortion is the oldest, and until recently the most dangerous, method of human fertility control throughout much of the world. Because of the increased distribution of modern contraceptives, the relative importance of abortion has diminished in some countries and has been superseded by voluntary sterilization and oral contraceptives.

Approximately 40 million abortions take place annually throughout the world; half of these are illegal and now represent a leading cause of death among women of childbearing age. In the Middle East and other areas of the world where family planning services are scarce, or where there is a lack of awareness and motivation regarding fertility regulation, health providers believe that the medical complications of illegal abortions are reaching epidemic dimensions (Johns Hopkins University, 1980).

The incidence of abortion is expected to escalate in the Middle East and other developing areas as a result of the following factors:

(1) Increasing preference for smaller families.
(2) A lack of effective family planning services for high-risk and vulnerable segments of the population.

In 1972 initial results on induced abortion from a 1-year study in one village in Egypt revealed that, at the start of the study, about 55 % of the women of childbearing age in the village were currently married, not sterile and not pregnant. Of these approximately 25 % became pregnant in the course of the study. About 25 % of the pregnancies resulted in abortions, of which approximately 20 % clearly were induced (about 5 % of all pregnancies). Although government family planning services are offered in this village, 30 % of the women reported they were unaware of the existence of such services (Foda *et al.*, 1972).

(3) An increase in the number of women of childbearing age and high birth rates in the Middle East.

In 1975, in Iran, the estimated crude birth and death rates were 45 and 14 per thousand, respectively, with an estimated natural increase in population of 3.1 % per year. Of this population, 47 % are aged 15 years or younger and 5 % are over 65. In Egypt the estimated crude birth and death rates in 1973 were 35 and 14–15 per thousand, respectively, with a growth rate of 2.0–2.1 %. During 1980, the crude birth rate rose to 40 per thousand with a resulting increase in the population growth rate. In Turkey, the crude birth and death rates for 1974 were estimated at about 37 and 12 per thousand, respectively, with a natural increase in population of 2.5 %. The vital rates for Tunisia, which has had enforced liberalization of abortions since 1973, are 37 per thousand for birth rate and 12 per thousand for death rate (in 1973) with a natural increase in population of 2.5 % per year. The annual crude birth rate in Morocco is around 45 and the natural growth rate is around 2.8 % per year (World Abortion Trends, 1979).

These nations all have a relatively young population with high fertility and relatively high, although decreasing, mortality. Population growth rates range from 2.5 % to 3.5 % per year except for Kuwait, which has substantial immigration, with an annual growth rate of +3.5 %.

(4) Social and economic factors, including a shift from rural to urban communities, high unemployment and other factors which lower the

perceived value of large extended families, may contribute to greater abortion demand (Tietze, 1983).

Abortion status in the Middle East *vs.* developed countries

The status of induced abortion ranges from complete restriction to elective abortion at the request of the pregnant woman. As of mid-1982, about two-thirds of the world's population lived in countries that permitted medically induced abortion on request or under a broad range of social conditions. Between 1965 and 1980, 40 countries extended the grounds for legal abortion while four other countries liberalized their abortion policies and later made them more restrictive: Israel, post-revolutionary Iran, New Zealand and the United States of America. The same situation occurred in four countries in Eastern Europe. Most of the countries that permit abortion under a broad range of conditions are located in Asia, Europe and North America (Cates and Grimes, 1981). In Egypt the present law demands the approval of two physicians to end a pregnancy for medical reasons that carry grave risk to the life of the expectant mother. In a study conducted in Alexandria, Egypt, the most common indication for therapeutic induced abortion was cardiovascular disease, but the number of cases quoted was insignificant (Toppozada *et al.*, 1980).

In countries with few restrictions, the distribution, quality and cost of abortion services are generally determined by government policy-makers and health administrators; e.g. in the United States financial assistance is largely unavailable to low-income women, and other restrictions, such as parental consent and mandatory waiting periods, restrict access to medical abortion services. Almost a third of American women live in counties where legal abortion services are not available (Alan Guttmacher Institute, 1982).

Major reasons advocated for less restrictive legislation concerning induced abortion are:

(1) public health, to combat illegal abortion and its associated morbidity and mortality;
(2) social justice, to give the poor access to abortion services previously available to the rich; and
(3) women's rights, to secure the claimed right of all women to control their own bodies.

Only a few countries, such as Singapore, Tunisia and, more recently, China, have adopted non-restrictive abortion policies to curb population growth. In countries where restrictive laws are enforced, women have not been discouraged from seeking abortion by other means, resorting to various methods of self-induced abortions and/or abortion by untrained, illegal practitioners. In Rumania, following passage of a more restrictive law in 1966, abortion-related deaths rose seven-fold over a decade and illegal abortions were obtained as often as legal ones (Tietze, 1983).

Opposition to the liberalization of abortion laws has been the tradition of conservatism based on moral and religious grounds. The Roman Catholic

Church is the strongest opponent, as are the fundamentalist Protestants, Muslims and Orthodox Jews. Over the last few years the highest abortion rates in the world appear to have been in Italy, Portugal and Uruguay. Most of the abortions in these three countries were illegal at the time. (Italy liberalized its abortion law in May 1978.) In Austria, Japan and the Soviet Union, where abortion is legal, more than one in two pregnancies end in abortion. In the middle range are Argentina, Bulgaria, Cuba, Hungary, Israel, Romania and Yugoslavia, with one abortion for every three pregnancies (Slater *et al.*, 1978). Countries with lower abortion rates of approximately one in four pregnancies include Brazil, East Germany, Finland, Poland, Sweden and the United States (Tietze, 1983). In Jordan 31.7% of all obstetric and gynecologic admissions are abortion cases. In Cairo University 50% of the Maternity Hospital budget is spent on abortions (induced or spontaneous). Of all women admitted to the Obstetrics and Gynecology Department, 35.5% had induced abortions (Foda *et al.*, 1972; Kamal *et al.*, 1972). In Shatby Hospital of the University of Alexandria, Egypt, the ratio of abortion to total admission in 10 years (1962–71) was 1 : 3.88 and the ratio of abortion to delivery in the same period was 1 : 1.86. Abortion accounted for 52.6% of all operations performed in the hospital (Shatby Maternity Hospital Annual Reports, 1978). In 1967 the incidence of both illegal and spontaneous abortions admitted in Ain Shams University Hospital in Cairo, Egypt, was 500 for every 1000 livebirths (Kamal *et al.*, 1972); while in Alexandria University Hospital in 1971 it was 588.2 per 1000 livebirths (Kamel *et al.*, 1974). In Kuwait, in the late 1960s, there were nine legal abortions among 32 000 deliveries. In Turkey the induced abortion ratio in 1968 was 38 per 100 livebirths (Bertan, 1975). In rural Egypt there is one illegal abortion for every 75 living children, while in urban parts of Egypt there is one for every 35 (Toppozada *et al.*, 1980). Criminal abortions account for 25% of all abortions in Cairo, Egypt (Suliman, 1979) and 16.4% of all abortions in Turkey (Bertan, 1975).

As a result of the restrictive status of abortion laws in most of the Middle East, physicians perform illegal abortions in private clinics and hospitals. In Egypt physicians in large medical centers induce abortions for women who have become pregnant with intrauterine contraceptive devices (IUCDs) *in situ*, although if prosecuted and convicted they could receive sentences of life imprisonment (Toppozada *et al.*, 1980). In a Turkish survey, 211 women reported a total of 462 induced abortions, 64% of which had been performed in physicians' offices and 14% in hospitals. Performing illegal abortions in this region of the world is a major source of income for some physicians and midwives. Consequently, some may have been opposed to the dissemination and use of effective contraceptive methods (Bertan, 1975; Tezcan *et al.*, 1980).

A study of three major hospitals in Cairo and Alexandria, Egypt, from 1965 to 1969, showed that between 496 and 575 women were admitted with abortion complications for every 1000 women admitted in labor. Also, a 1967 survey of over 3800 teachers in Alexandra reported that 34% of the women who had ever been pregnant had had at least one spontaneous or induced abortion, and over 23% of all pregnancies ended in abortion (Kamel *et al.*, 1970). In Iran a study for analysis of rural and urban age-specific fertility rates and contraceptive use found that 25 000–33 000 abortions were induced in 1966 in Tehran, or one abortion for every three to five livebirths (Johns Hopkins University, 1980). In the last decade an increasing number of women in the Middle East have relied on abortion to prevent an unwanted birth. In Tunisia, because of legalized abortion status, it is used basically as a back-up in cases of contraceptive failure (Tunisia: Office National du Planning Familial et de la Population, 1979). Turkish women are believed to have the highest prevalence of illegal abortion in the Middle East because effective family planning methods are not immediately available and the desired family size is small (Tezcan et al., 1980; Tezcan and Omran, 1981). In other Middle Eastern countries, such as Saudi Arabia, Afghanistan and Bahrain, there is no mention of abortion in their statute books, so practice of such is presumed to be illegal.

In the United States the number of illegal induced abortions probably declined during the 1960s as more effective contraceptive methods were used by a growing number of couples, and as surgical sterilization became increasingly available and acceptable by both males and females. The decline of illegal abortion was balanced by the progressive liberalization of abortion laws. From 1970 onward there was a precipitous drop in the number of deaths related to illegally induced abortions (60 % fewer in New York City after 9 months), a 5 % decline in the birth rate, and a 4 % decline in illegitimate births (Pakter and Nelson, 1971). Also, the number of 'spontaneous' incomplete abortions was reduced by 52 %, confirming the hypothesis that a large number of incomplete abortions are induced (Cates et al., 1978; Cates and Grimes, 1981).

Abortion statistics in England and Wales demonstrated dramatic effects of the passage of the Abortion Act of 1967, in that the number of legal abortions performed on resident women increased during the first 12 months about three-fold. From 1967 to 1976 the number of abortions declined slightly, then rose in 1980; in 1981 the increase stopped. Both rates and ratios are substantially lower in England and Wales than in the United States, or in some of the countries of Northern and Eastern Europe (Bone, 1982; Tietze, 1983).

Demographic characteristics of patients in selected countries in the region

Most Middle Eastern women who obtain abortions desire to limit family size. Women most likely to terminate their pregnancies are married, over age 25, with three or more living children. The prevalence of abortion increases with age. In a 1976 survey of 1459 Lebanese women, 20–24 years of age, it was reported that 14.4 % of their pregnancies had ended in abortion, while for women aged 40–44 the rate was 60 %. Pregnancy and illegal abortion among unmarried women seem to be relatively rare (World Abortion Trends, 1979; World Health Organization, 1978).

The proportion of women under age 20 obtaining legal abortions increased to more than 30 % in Norway, England, New Zealand, Scotland, Canada and the United States. This increase could be observed in the majority of countries, but the proportion dropped to 18 % in Sweden, and the lowest proportion of such young women are now reported from Tunisia and Japan. In Tunisia the percentage of legal abortions per age group in 1978 was 2.5 % for age 19 or less, 16.5 % for 20–24, 50.5 % for 25–34, 20.0 % for 35–39, and 10.5 % for age 40 or more. With regard to parity, the percentage of legal abortions by 1978 was 7.1 % for para. 0, 40.3 % for para. 1 to 3; 16.9 % for para. 4 and 35.7 % for para. 5 or more, indicating higher parity than in other countries with legalized abortion. Three in five women who obtained a legal abortion in 1976 had had four or more prior births (Tietze, 1983).

In the Middle East, abortion is more common in urban areas and among the better educated. In Lebanon the issue of whether a woman is Muslim or Christian may be less important in determining abortion practice than her education level and area of residence. Among Muslims in a 1961 study, over 30 % of educated urban women reported having had induced abortion, compared to 13 % of uneducated urban women and 2 % of uneducated rural women. Similar differences were seen among Christian women (Nazer, 1972; Toppozada *et al.*, 1980). Regarding socioeconomic classes it is generally agreed that abortion is more common among women in upper and middle classes than in the lower classes. In 1970 and 1971 women in Lebanon, Iran and Turkey were surveyed as part of a World Health Organization collaborative study on family formation patterns and health. In each country, middle-class women reported a greater percentage of pregnancies ending in abortion than did lower-class women (Toppozada *et al.*, 1980; Toppozada and Toppozada, 1972).

An epidemiologic study in Alexandria, Egypt, used the prospective approach with a retrospective case control design and collected data on abortion for the 3-year period from 1974 to 1977 (Toppozada *et al.*, 1980). The great majority of women who had had abortions were urban dwellers and only approximately 4 % of the study group were Christians. Approximately 99 % were currently married, only a few cases were pregnant out-of-wedlock and a minority were divorced or widowed. Also, there was a direct relationship between the education level of the woman and the rate of abortion. The women who had criminal abortions were significantly older, but the number of pregnancies and livebirths was not significantly different between cases of criminal and spontaneous abortions in the two groups (prospective and retrospective).

Since many women in developing countries who seek abortions already have all the children they want, expanded voluntary sterilization services may provide an alternative.

SOME SEQUELAE OF ABORTION

Complications resulting from induced abortion

Induced abortion, at any stage of gestation, exposes a woman to the risk of complications that can vary, depending on the cicumstances under which the abortion is performed. Complications are either minor or major with occasional fatal outcome. Early complications may be immediate, as those occurring during the procedure or within a few hours after its completion, or may occur within 1 month (Tietze, 1983). Late complications occur more than 1 month after the procedure.

Fertility may be compromised and maternal morbidity increased by serious early complications such as: (1) perforation of the uterus with or without injury to intestines or other organs; (2) major hemorrhage; (3) laceration of the cervix; (4) severe disturbances of blood coagulation; and (5) untoward effects of general or local anesthesia. The most frequent delayed complications are: (1) retention of fragments of placenta resulting in postabortal bleeding; (2) infection, ranging from mild endometritis and more severe forms of pelvic inflammatory disease to generalized peritonitis and septicemia; (3) venous thrombophlebitis resulting in pulmonary embolism or infarction; and (4) postabortal depression.

A clearcut causal relationship between the abortion and the woman's inability to conceive or to produce viable offspring may be evident:

(1) Sterility can result from hysterectomy performed because of major hemorrhage in the course of another abortion procedure; the incidence of these events increase with age.

(2) Secondary sterility can be the late result of pelvic inflammatory disease (PID), which is a not-uncommon complication following abortions in non-medical settings, as well as legal abortions. Also, Westrom (1980) in Sweden suggested an increased incidence of ectopic pregnancy following legal abortion complicated by PID, on the order of one per 3000 total abortions, added to an expected frequency of one ectopic per 150 pregnancies approximately (Tietze, 1983). Having had one ectopic pregnancy reduced a woman's monthly probability of conception by about one-half if the other tube is intact and by even more if both tubes have been damaged by the PID.

(3) A third mechanism by which an abortion can impair a woman's chances of producing viable offspring is immunization of a woman with Rh-negative factor by red blood cells from a fetus with Rh-positive factor entering her bloodstream at the time of the procedure. The risk is less in early pregnancy, but increases with the duration of gestation. Rh-immunization may result in severe, often fatal, damage to the newborn. It can'be prevented with Rh-immune globulin injection at the time of the abortion to all Rh-negative women (15 % in the US) unless the partner is known to be Rh-negative also (Tietze, 1983; Toppozada et al., 1980).

There is emphasis on damage to the cervix during dilatation, or damage to the uterine wall resulting in intrauterine adhesions (Asherman syndrome). Investigations regarding future childbearing after an induced abortion concluded that the possible adverse effects are secondary sterility, ectopic pregnancy, spontaneous abortion, premature delivery and low infant birth weight. These studies were reviewed and debated by Hogue and associates (1982).

Complications resulting from illegal abortion

Worldwide, the most frequent complication of legal and illegal abortion is incomplete abortion or retained products of conception, which requires evacuation of the uterus. The most frequent major complications of illegal abortion are pelvic infection, hemorrhage and shock. Another very frequently reported complication is trauma to pelvic organs, such as cervical lacerations, uterine perforation and damage to the bladder and intestines. In some developing countries of the Middle East, tetanus complication is sporadically fatal.

The types of drugs and techniques used to attempt illegal abortion are many, ranging from herbal teas to modern surgery. Potassium permanganate tablets and other chemical substances inserted into the cervical os can cause chemical burns and bleeding, and may even lead to the formation of bladder or rectal fistulae. Abdominal massage by granny-midwives, or Dayas, can cause internal bleeding and organ damage (Johns Hopkins University, 1980). Mechanical methods, such as insertion of a catheter or a twig of a plant, may lead to uterine, bladder or intestinal perforation and subsequent peritonitis. Other non-medical methods to induce abortion include eating or drinking quinine or other chemicals that can lead to poisoning, renal failure or intense vomiting, causing dehydration and eventually death unless proper therapy is instituted (Johns Hopkins University, 1980).

Maternal mortality

It is difficult to assess the number of deaths caused by illegal abortion in the Middle East. Based on a computer model simulating reproductive events, Tietze (1983) has estimated that, where most abortions are either self-induced or performed by unskilled persons in areas with poor medical care systems, mortality from illegal abortion may be as high as 1000 deaths per 100 000 illegal procedures. In most countries, mortality — while still high — is probably no more than 50–100 deaths per 100 000 illegal abortions (Tietze, 1983).

The mortality rate from illegally induced abortions in Alexandria, Egypt, was 135 per 100 000. This can be compared to the mortality rate in the US before legalization of abortion, which was 100 per 100 000 ('ı oppozada *et al.*, 1980).

Since hospital admissions for abortion complications include women with either spontaneous or illegal induced abortions, and since spontaneous abortion is less likely to be life-threatening than illegal abortion, these hospital mortality ratios underestimate mortality from illegal induced abortions (Tables 2.1 and 2.2). Hospitals in India have very high ratios for complications of illegal abortions ranging from 8 to 307 deaths per 1000 admissions (Tietze *et al.*, 1976).

Mortality from legal abortion is much lower than mortality from illegal abortion, as is seen in Tunisia. In 1977 the United States Center for Disease Control (CDC) reported a mortality ratio for legal abortion of 1.4 deaths per 100 000 legal abortions.

Table 2.1 Deaths in hospitals attributed to complications of induced and spontaneous abortion as a proportion of maternal deaths in hospitals

	Maternal deaths attributed to abortion complications	
	No.	*Percentage*
Iran, 1963–69, Pahlavi University, Tehran	7	7.3
Iraq, 1964–70, Baghdad	5	9.4

Table 2.2 Deaths in hospitals attributed to complications of induced or spontaneous abortion as a proportion of all hospital admissions for complications of abortion

	Admissions for abortion complications (No.)	*Deaths due to abortion complications (No.)*	*Deaths per 1000 admissions for abortion complications (No.)*
Egypt			
1971–73, Kasr El Aini, Cairo	736	0	0
1969, Kasr El Aini, Cairo	1620	1	0.6
1973, Tanta Univ. Hosp.	913	8	8.8
1973–74, El Galaa Hosp., Cairo	388	1	2.6
Kuwait			
1973–77, Kuwait Mater. Hosp.	21018	2	0.1
Lebanon			
1961–71, Amer. Univ. Hosp., Beirut	3190	15	4.7
Sudan			
1974, three hosp., Khartoum	1191	0	0

FAMILY PLANNING AND ABORTION

Induced abortion and family planning share a common goal of preventing unwanted or unplanned pregnancy. There is a high correlation between abortion experience and contraceptive experience in populations for whom family planning methods and abortion services are available and in which some couples have tried to regulate the number and spacing of their children. In such populations women who have practiced contraception are more likely to have had abortions than those who have not, and women who have had abortions are more likely to use contraceptives than women without a history of pregnancy termination (Tietze, 1983).

Among women who do not want to become pregnant, but not all of whom practice contraception, the abortion ratio tends to be high. Women who practice contraception consistently and effectively experience fewer unwanted pregnancies over a period of time and, therefore, have a lower abortion rate than those who practice contraception ineffectively or not at all (Gaslonde Sainz, 1976). A change in the abortion rate may be associated with a change in the pregnancy rate either in the same direction or in the opposite direction. Some factors and variables affecting these rates include distribution of the population by age (15 – 44) and marital status; the proportion of unmarried, sexually active women; the proportion of sexually active women who intend to become pregnant and deliver a baby; the contraceptive behavior of sexually active women who do not desire conception, including use or neglect of contraceptive methods; and the level of contraceptive circumspection (Tietze, 1983).

Abortion alone is an inefficient method of fertility regulation, but it is adequate as a back-up method in conjunction with the use of contraceptives. It has been shown conclusively that reliance on barrier methods, with early abortion as a back-up, is the safest and reversible regimen of fertility regulation at any age (Tietze *et al.*, 1976; Tietze, 1983).

It has been advocated that to achieve the two-child family average needed for population stabilization, some reliance on abortion would probably be required, since present contraceptive methods are neither totally effective nor universally available. Reducing fertility from an average of seven births per woman to an average of two, in the absence of contraceptives, would require an average of nine to ten abortions per woman. Studies conducted in several countries demonstrate that, while countries with falling birth rates can reduce abortion rates through intensive family planning programs, only the universal use of a perfect contraceptive would largely eliminate the need for abortion services. Also, there is an indication that the availability of abortion services as a crisis intervention may reinforce contraceptive practice. Women who have had an abortion are more likely to practice contraception than are other women. Even in countries where abortion is illegal, clinics and hospitals have seen increased contraceptive acceptance through family planning counseling programs for clients admitted for abortion-related complications. This positive association between abortion and contraception is most evident where legal abortion services are part of a comprehensive family planning program offering a full range of contraceptives and voluntary sterilization. In three Sudanese hospitals over 2700 women hospitalized for abortion complications were asked about contraceptive use before abortion and 2–4 weeks afterwards; 10% had used contraception before, compared with 47% afterward. Better counseling, provision of a larger supply of contraceptives and better follow-up may encourage even more women to accept contraceptives after abortion and to continue using them (Johns Hopkins University, 1980).

In a retrospective and prospective abortion study (Toppozada *et al.*, 1980), it was demonstrated that 39.99% of the prospective abortees accepted family planning after abortion and the acceptability was much higher among induced cases (80.95%) than among spontaneous abortees (38.62%). The reason given most frequently (72.34%) for accepting family planning was to achieve the ideal family size. Induced abortees were more likely to use a contraceptive method immediately after the abortion than spontaneous abortees. Oral contraceptives were the most accepted method (72.54%). Most cases

20

(66.18%) received their knowledge and family planning education from the medical team while they were in the hospital. In the retrospective group, 31.52% practised family planning after the abortion. Oral contraceptives were chosen by 62.80% of the acceptors and, on an average, the chosen methods were used for 2.13 ± 1.64 years after the abortion. If a woman is to be fully protected from the risk of another unwanted pregnancy, methods of contraception must be made available before hospital discharge.

SPONTANEOUS ABORTION: IS IT ACTUALLY INDUCED?

Accurate statistics are unavailable on the number of illegal induced abortions performed throughout the world. Because of the clandestine nature of abortions, public health workers are unable to measure their incidence directly. Therefore, epidemiologic studies of illegal abortions rely on indirect methods of ascertainment. These methods include: (1) use of vital statistics to compare vital events before and after liberalization of abortion laws; (2) use of hospital-based abortion morbidity and mortality data; (3) use of reproductive mathematical models to determine pregnancy outcome; and (4) use of reproductive behavior survey data.

Of 5031 abortion cases studied retrospectively, only 405 admitted having had at least one criminally induced abortion, a proportion of 8.05% of the sample (Toppozada *et al.*, 1980). The most frequent diagnosis in the prospective cases was inevitable abortion (41.58%). Incomplete abortion was encountered in 28.76% of the cases, while 22.34% were admitted as threatening abortions. Knowledge of the incidence of abortions, and whether they are spontaneous or induced, is of value in the study of fertility and other biological variables in any community. Induced abortion rates vary widely among countries and regions, reflecting differences in premarital sexual behavior, age at marriage, desired family size, availability and access to family planning services, and use of contraceptives for spacing pregnancies or for permanent fertility regulation. Estimates of induced abortions per year worldwide range from 30 to 55 million, roughly half of which are illegally induced. Even the incidence of spontaneous abortion during the first trimester is not registered; since some women conceive and abort unnoticed, its incidence is likely to be greater than the present rate of 15–20%. Most septic and incomplete abortions are thought to be criminally induced, but many illegally induced abortions show no signs or symptoms of infections (World Abortion Trends, 1979).

CONCLUSIONS

A major cause of death among women of reproductive age in the Middle East is illegally induced abortion. Complications of the procedure account for 4–70% of maternal deaths in hospitals and an unknown number of additional deaths outside hospitals. The incidence of abortion seems to be increasing as more women try to avoid unwanted births and keep family size small. To reduce mortality due to illegal abortion and to improve maternal and infant health, different approaches are suggested, as follows:

(1) Encouraging the use of contraception rather than abortion, by educational programs aimed especially at the first encounter when women are in hospitals for health care, or by an outreach program contacting the vulnerable segment of the population and/or by mass media. Emphasis must be given to the fact that risks from modern contraceptives are much less than the risks from illegal abortion. The intrauterine contraceptive device program is very successful during the immediate post-reproductive event period when women are highly motivated. Male education is a very important factor in enhancing knowledge, attitude and practice in family planning, because husbands in the Middle Eastern countries are the ultimate heads of families and have the final word on fertility regulation. Correcting false notions regarding contraceptives, and increasing the emphasis on the concept of spacing births rather than on preventing conception, may lead to better understanding, communication and acceptance of family planning.

(2) Individual counseling about proper use, use-effectiveness and side-effects of various contraceptive methods. It is also recommended to introduce abortion as a back-up method in case of contraceptive failure so that the woman will feel secure and not resort to illegal induced abortion with its risks.

(3) Increasing the availability of health services for all women, especially those with high-risk status, to be provided during pre-conception, inter-conception and post-conception periods with emphasis on nutrition, immunization, fertility regulation, health education, preventive medicine and child care.

(4) Modification of present abortion laws in some countries in the region, either to complete legalization, as in Tunisia, or to allow legal abortion for medical/social reasons encompassing a multiplicity of conditions so as to be flexible and reasonable. This would allow medically trained practitioners to perform these abortions, thus lowering health risks.

(5) Improved clinical management of abortion complications, especially septic cases which require prompt care and optimum treatment (evacuation of uterus, antibiotic treatment and monitoring of fluid and electrolyte balance).

The levels and trends of fertility regulation are determined by broad social forces. These include antinatalist and pronatalist government policies, the response to which may be facilitated or obstructed by a greater or lesser availability of abortion. The final decision is in the hands of the governments.

Acknowledgments

My gratitude to Dr Ashraf A. Ismail, Egyptian Ministry of Health, for his great help, and to Ms Kathy Lianza and Ms Lynn Rudloff for their sincere effort in typing and proof-reading this chapter.

References

Alan Guttmacher Institute (1982). Estimated numbers of legal abortions by woman's race, age, parity, marital status, prior induced abortions, weeks of gestation, and type of procedure, prepared by S. K. Henshaw

Bchir, M. and Charfeddine, A. (1978). *Évolution des principales caractéristiques démographiques des contraceptrices au courant de la trienne 1974–1976.* (Tunis: Office National du Planning Familial et de la Population)

Bertan, M. (Hacetep University, Ankara, Turkey) (1975). Task force on sequelae and complications of induced abortion meeting, Geneva, 27–30 October 1975. WHO Mimeograph

Bone, M. (1982). The 'Pill scare' and fertility in England and Wales. *IPPF Med. Bull.*, **16**(4), 2–4

Cates, W., Jr. and Grimes, D. A. (1981). Morbidity and mortality of abortion in the United States. In Hodgson, J. E (ed.) *Abortion and Sterilization: Medical and Social Aspects.* pp. 155–80. (London: Academic Press)

Cates, W., Jr., Smith, J. C., Rachat, R. W., Patterson, J. E. and Dolman, A. (1978). Assessment of surveillance and vital statistics data for monitoring abortion mortality, United States, 1972–1975. *Am. J. Epidemiol.*, **108**, 200–6

Charfeddine, A. (1980). Évolution récente de Programme National de Planning Familial. *Rev. Tunisienne Ét. Popul.*, **1**, 105–30

Foda, M. S., Darwish, N. H., Shafeek, M. A., Osman, E. and Nomrosi, M. (1972). Abortion in Egypt. In Nazer, I. R. (ed.) *Induced Abortion: A Hazard to Public Health?* p. 122. (Beirut: International Planned Parenthood Federation)

Gaslonde Sainz, S. (1976). Abortion research in Latin America. *Stud. Fam. Plann.*, **7**, 211–17

Hogue, C. J. R., Cates, W., Jr. and Tietze, C. (1982). The effects of induced abortion on subsequent reproduction. *Epidemiol. Rev.*, **4**, 66–94

Johns Hopkins University: Population Information Program (1980). Complications of abortion in developing countries. *Popul. Rep.* (*F*), **7**, 105–55

Kalkili, A. (Jordanian Mofti) (1974). In Nazer, I. (ed.) *Islam and Abortion.* p. 77. (IPPF Meeting in Rabat, Morocco), Arabia

Kamal, I., Ghoneim, M. A., Talaat, M., Abdallah, M. and Eid, M. (1972). An attempt at estimating the magnitude and probable incidence of induced abortion in the UAR. In Nazer, I. (ed.) *Induced Abortion: A Hazard to Public Health?* p. 106. (Beirut: International Planned Parenthood Federation)

Kamel, N., Kamel, S. and Abul-Einin, M. (1974). Abortion and abortees in 1971 at Shatby Maternity Hospital. *Bull. High Inst. Publ. Health Alexandria*, **IV**, 137–55

Kamel, W. H., Wahdan, M. H. and Kamel, N. M. (1970). Family planning stu-ies – the teacher's survey. *Egyptian Popul. Fam. Plann. Rev.*, **3**, 17

Law No. 44 of 1979 (1979). Modification of some bilaws of the civil personal conditions law, Cairo

Nazer, I. R. (ed.) (1972). *Induced Abortion: A Hazard to Public Health?* (Beirut: International Planned Parenthood Federation)

Pakter, J. and Nelson, F. (1971). Abortion in New York City: the first nine months. *Fam. Plann. Perspect.*, **3**, 5

Population Crisis Committee (1979). World abortion trends. *Population*, **9**, 1–6

Shatby Maternity Hospital Annual Reports, 1962–71 (1978). (H. K. Toppozada, ed.). Alexandria University Press, Alexandria, Egypt

Slater, P., Weiner, D. and Davies, A. M. (1978). Illegal abortion in Israel. *Israel Law Rev.*, **13**, 411–16

Suliman, N. H. (1979). Abortion in Egypt. Population Studies. Issued by the Egyptian Supreme Council for Population and Family Planning, **49**, 14–16

Tezcan, S. and Omran, A. R. (1981). Prevalence and reporting of induced abortion in Turkey: two survey techniques. *Stud. Fam. Plann.*, **12**, 262–71

Tezcan, S., Carpenter-Yaman, C. E. and Fisek, N. H. (1980). *Abortion in Turkey.* (Ankara, Turkey: Hacettepe University Institute of Community Medicine)

Tietze, C. (1983). *Induced Abortion: 1983*, 5th edn. (New York: Population Council)

Tietze, C., Bongaarts, J. and Schearer, B. (1976). Mortality associated with the control of fertility. *Fam. Plann. Perspect.*, **8**, 6–14

Toppozada, H. K. and Toppozada, M. K. (1972). Induced abortion in private cases in Alexandria. In Nazer, I. (ed.) *Induced Abortion: A Hazard to Public Health?* pp. 168–77. (Beirut: International Planned Parenthood Federation)

Toppozada, H. K., Rizk, M. A., Abul-Einin, M. A., Medhat, I., Kamel, N. M., Kamel, S. M. and Hussein, M. H. (1980). Epidemiology of abortion in Alexandria. *Alexandria Med. J.*, **26**(1, 2)

Tunisia: Office National du Planning Familial et de la Population (1979). *Statistiques de Planning Familial*, no. 17, supplemented by unpublished data for 1979

Weström, L. (1980). Incidence, prevalence, and trends of acute pelvic inflammatory disease and its consequences in industrialized countries. *Am. J. Obstet. Gynecol.*, **138**, 880–92

World Health Organization (1978). *Induced Abortion.* (Geneva: Technical Report Series, no. 623)

Bibliography

Berelson, B. (1979). Romania's 1966 antiabortion decree: the demographic experience of the first decade. *Pop. Stud.*, **33**, 209–22

Berger, G. S., Tietze, C., Pakter, J. and Katz, S. H. (1974). Maternal mortality associated with legal abortion in New York State: July 1, 1970 – June 30, 1972. *Obstet. Gynecol.*, **43**, 315–26

Bongaarts, J. and Tietze, C. (1977). The efficiency of menstrual regulation as a method of fertility control. *Stud. Fam. Plann.*, **8**, 268–72

Brewer, C. (1977). Incidence of postabortion psychosis: a prospective study. *Br. Med. J.*, **1** (6059), 476–7

Chung, C. S., Steinhoff, P. G. and Smith, R. G. (1981). Effects of Induced Abortion on Subsequent Reproductive Functions and Pregnancy Outcome. Final Report, Contract No. (N01-HD-62801) (Honolulu: University of Hawaii)

Fortney, J. A., Miller, E. R. and Kessel, E. (1977). Competing risks of unnecessary procedures and complications. *Stud. Fam. Plann.*, **8**, 257–62

Harlap, S. and Davies, A. M. (1975). Late sequalae of induced abortion: complications and outcome of pregnancy and labour. *Am. J. Epidemiol.*, **102**, 217

Harlap, S., Shiono, P. H., Ramcharan, S., Berendes, H. and Pellegrin, F. (1979). A prospective study of spontaneous fetal losses after induced abortions. *N. Engl. J. Med.*, **301** (13), 677–81

Kimball, A. M., Hallum, A. V. and Cates, W., Jr. (1978). Deaths caused by pulmonary thromboembolism after legally induced abortion. *Am. J. Obstet. Gynecol.*, **132**, 169–73

Nazer, I. (1977). A study on the trends in abortion practice in Tunisia since the legalization of abortion on socio-economic grounds. Monograph, p. 7

Naziha Lakehal – Ayat. (1979). *La femme Tunisienne et sa place dans le droit positif.* (Tunis: Dar El Amal)

Pantelakis, S. N., Papadimitriou, G. C. and Doxiadis, S. A. (1973). Influence of induced and spontaneous abortions on the outcome of subsequent pregnancies. *Am. J. Obstet. Gynecol.*, **116**, 799

Potts, M., Diggory, P. and Peel, J. (1977). *Abortion.* (Cambridge and New York: Cambridge University Press)

Selim, A. M. (Grand Egyptian Mofti) (1972). Fatwa given on 27.1.1937 No. 43. In Superior Council of Family Planning (ed.) *Religion's Idea of Family Planning.* (Cairo: Abram Commercial Printers)

Tietze, C. and Lewit, S. (1972). Joint program for the study of abortion (JPSA): early medical complications of legal abortion. *Stud. Fam. Plann.*, **3**, 97–122 (supplemented by unpublished data)

World Health Organization (1970). *Spontaneous and Induced Abortion.* (Geneva: Technical Report Series, No. 461)

World Health Organization: Task Force on Sequelae of Abortion (1979). Gestation, birthweight and spontaneous abortion in pregnancy after induced abortion. *Lancet*, **1** (8108), 142–5

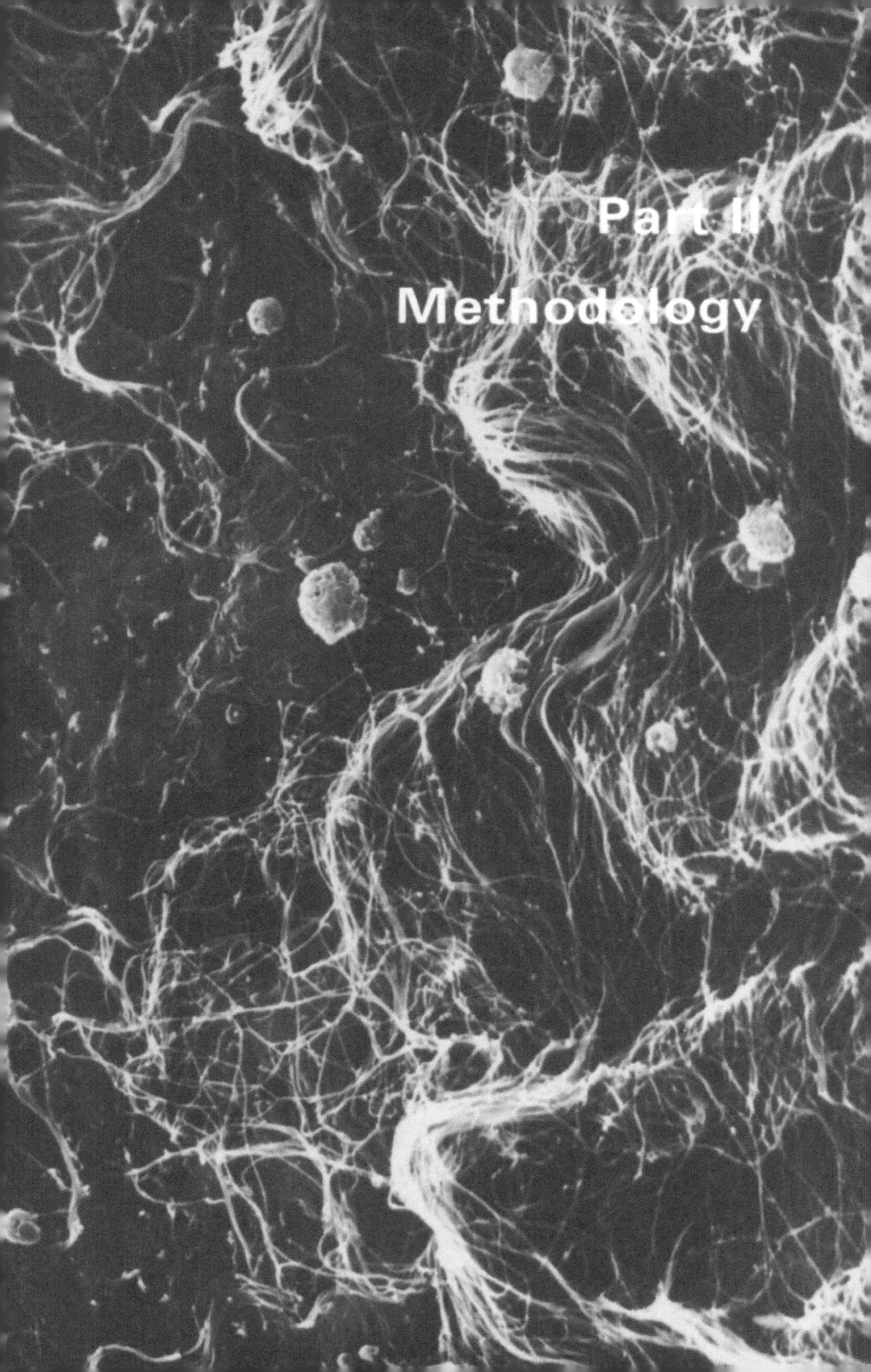

Part II
Methodology

3
Mid-trimester abortion using extraovular normal saline

H. ABRAMOVICI, A. ROFE, J. ATAD and J. H. FAKTOR

The evacuation of a large uterus is a dangerous procedure with complication rates three to four times higher than uterine evacuation in the first trimester (Danforth, 1982). Fifteen percent of abortions performed in the USA between 1972 and 1975 were mid-trimester abortions, which accounted for almost 60 % of abortion-related maternal death (Cates *et al.*, 1977).

In an effort to lower the complication rates, many methods have been tried, differing according to the success rates but having in common a high rate of incidents, accidents and complications. The methods available to terminate a mid-trimester pregnancy or a mid-trimester missed abortion utilize various approaches, as shown below.

The vaginal route

Intravaginal administration of prostaglandins PGE_2 or $PG_{2\alpha}$ suppositories can induce evacuation of a large uterus with a large degree of success. The method is simple, relatively safe but the drug-related side effects of pros- taglandins (nausea, vomiting, diarrhea, bronchospasm, etc.) are not in- frequent (Schulman *et al.*, 1974; Lauersen *et al.*, 1975).

Dilatation and curettage or vacuum aspiration may be the solution to the problem of a large uterus between 12 and 15 weeks only. However, this procedure has an increased risk of uterine perforation, incomplete evacuation, infections, cervical damage, etc. (Lauersen, 1981; Cates *et al.*, 1979).

The extraovular route for administration of rivanol, hypertonic saline, prostaglandins or other drugs was described by Scandinavian and Japanese gynecologists. This route is quite simple and safe, but side effects related to the various drugs used for frequently encountered (Gustavii, 1974; Halbrecht and Blum, 1974; Wiqvist *et al.*, 1974; Shapiro, 1975).

The intra-amniotic route

This is the most widely used approach. It consists of amniocentesis and intra- amniotic instillation of pharmacological agents such as hypertonic glucose, urea, hypertonic saline, prostaglandins, etc. All these drugs injected into the amniotic sac are effective in producing abortion by different mechanisms. However, they tend to induce drug-related side effects which are characteristic according to the drug used: hypernatremia and consumption coagulopathy where hypertonic saline is used, gastrointestinal symptoms, uterine hypertonicity, bronchospasm where prostaglandins are administered, severe infection where hypertonic glucose is used, etc. (McDonald and Aaro, 1975; Berger *et al.*, 1975). In addition to these drug-related complications, there are difficulties related to the amniocentesis itself, especially in cases of obese women, anterior location of placenta or in mid-trimester missed abortion cases, where there is little or no fluid left in the amniotic cavity.

The parenteral route

Oral, intravenous or intramuscular prostaglandins or intravenous oxytocin are used to induce mid-trimester abortions as primary methods but are more frequently used in order to shorten the instillation–abortion time when other methods are used. The drug-related side effects are not infrequent.

The abdominal operative route

Hysterotomy or hysterectomy are rarely performed these days in order to evacuate a large uterus. These are surgical procedures associated with the relevant operative morbidity and mortality rates (Lauersen, 1981). They are recommended today only in cases where other methods have failed, when the woman wants to combine abortion with sterilization or when there is associated uterine or ovarian pathology – e.g. uterine fibroids, ovarian cysts or tumors.

Most of the complications in mid-trimester abortions have two main features:

(1) the drug-related side effects and complications;
(2) the difficulties and complications related to the needle penetration into the amniotic sac when the intra-amniotic route is used.

To avoid these two main sources of complications, we use normal saline (having no side effects), which is instilled, not intra-amniotically, but through the normal physiologic opening of the cervix into the extraovular space. This is done by using a specially designed double balloon catheter (Atad's Catheter, manufactured by Porges, France), which is introduced through the cervix to a depth of 10 cm into the extraovular space without rupturing the membranes (Fig. 3.1). The catheter is guided to the opposite side of the placental insertion. When the catheter is positioned and the two balloons are inflated (30 cm³ normal saline), one balloon occludes the external os and the other the internal os of the cervix, thus preventing leakage of the saline solution from the extraovular space through the cervix into the vagina (Rofe *et al.*, 1980; Abramovici *et al.*, 1981).

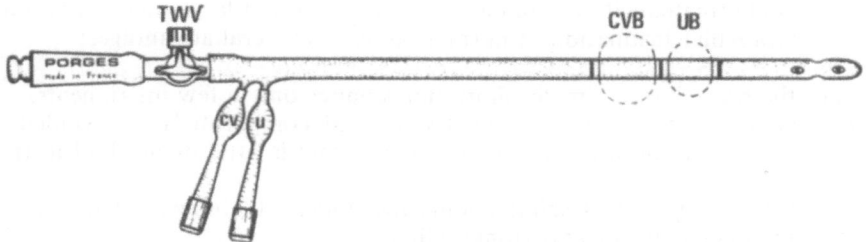

Fig. 3.1 Atad double balloon catheter for late interruption of pregnancy. Porges Art. No. 3710, 618, TWV: three way valve; CV: cervicovaginal valve; U: uterine valve; CVB: cervicovaginal balloon; UB: uterine balloon

In every case an ultrasonic examination should be performed prior to the procedure, in order to locate the placenta and to rule out placenta praevia, which is a contraindication to using this method. After positioning the catheter, 20 ml of normal saline for every week of gestational age is slowly instilled through the catheter into the extraovular space. At the end of the instillation process the proximal end of the catheter is occluded and taped to the patient's leg. After the procedure the patient is unrestricted in her activities until the onset of her contractions. The introduction of the catheter and the instillation of the saline and painless procedures. There is no need for anesthesia, analgesia or premedication. A few hours after the instillation of the normal saline, uterine contractions start and patients abort the fetus in an intact amniotic sac, including the placenta.

After the expulsion of the fetus and placenta, a gentle control curettage is performed in order to assure that the uterine cavity is empty. The day after the abortion the woman is discharged, and after a few days of rest she resumes her activities. All Rh-negative patients must receive an injection of $Rh_0(D)$ immune globulin within 72 h of the abortion. The mechanism of abortion by using this procedure is not fully understood. Endogenic prostaglandin studies performed in a few patients suggest that there is a marked rise in the level of prostaglandins immediately following the procedure. The mechanical separation of the ovum by the extraovular instillation of the normal saline induces an increase in local endogenous prostaglandins that is responsible for the onset of contractions.

Over 100 uterine evacuations of mid-trimester pregnancy were performed (54 cases of normal pregnancies and 48 cases of mid-trimester missed abortions). All patients aborted as a result of the procedure and the mean instillation-to-abortion interval was 30 h in the normal pregnancy group and 16 h in the missed abortion cases. Forty-eight percent of the patients in the normal pregnancy group, and 73 % of the patients in the missed abortion group, aborted during the first 24 h. There was no correlation between the parity or gestational age and the instillation–abortion time. The use of additional intravenous pitocin did not shorten the instillation-to-abortion interval. There was no maternal morbidity or complications during or following the procedure, except three cases of post-abortion endometritis sucessfully treated with antibiotics. The evacuation of large uterus by using the extraovular instillation of normal saline has several advantages:

(1)   the procedure is simple, short and requires only a few instruments;
(2)   amniocentesis with its related risks and complications is avoided – this is an important advantage when there is little or no fluid in the amniotic cavity;
(3)   the use of normal saline avoids the undesirable effects of oxytocin, prostaglandins or hypertonic saline.

The only contraindication to this procedure is in cases with central placenta praevia, because of the danger of severe bleeding. Patients proved by ultrasonography to have this condition should be aborted by other methods. The clinician must choose the method best suited to his patient and facilities, taking into account the patient's medical and gynecological state, as well as local conditions.

References

Abramovici, H., Rofe, A., Atad, J. and Lewin, A. (1981). Termination of mid-trimester missed abortion by extraovular instillation of normal saline. *Br. J. Obstet. Gynaecol.*, **88**, 931–3

Berger, G. S., Edelman, D. A. and Kerenyi, T. D. (1975). Oxytocin administration, instillation-to-abortion time and morbidity associated with saline instillation. *Am. J. Obstet. Gynecol.*, **121**, 941–6

Cates, W., Jr., Grimes, D. A. and Smith, J. C. (1977). The risk of dying from legal abortion in the United States, 1973–1975. *Int. J. Gynaecol. Obstet.*, **15**, 172–6

Cates, W., Jr., Schulz, K. F., Gold, J. and Tyler, W. C. (1979). Complications of surgical evacuation procedures for abortion after 12 weeks' gestation. In Zatuchni, I. G., Sciarra, J. J. and Speidel, J. (eds.) *Pregnancy Termination, Procedures, Safety and New Developments.* Chapter 26, pp. 206–16. (Hagerstown: Harper & Row)

Danforth, D. (1982). *Obstetrics and Gynecology*, 4th edn. p. 280. (Philadelphia: Harper & Row Publishers)

Gustavii, B. (1974). Intraamniotic and extraamniotic infection of sodium chloride solution: amniotic fluid salinity and abortifacient effect. *Am. J. Obstet. Gynecol.*, **118**, 218–22

Halbrecht, I. and Blum, M. (1974). Induction of midtrimester abortion by means of extra-amniotic infusion of an isotonic saline solution combined with intravenous oxytocin drip infusion. *Contraception*, **10**, 637–44

Lauersen, N. H. (1981). Spontaneous and therapeutic abortion. In Schaefer, G. and Graber, A. E. (eds.) *Complications in Obstetrics and Gynecologic Surgery.* p. 86. (Hagerstown: Harper & Row)

Lauersen, N. H., Secher, H. J. and Wilson, K. L. (1975). Midtrimester abortion induced by intravaginal administration of prostaglandin E_2 suppositories. *Am. J. Obstet. Gynecol.*, **122**, 947–54

McDonald, T. T. and Aaro, L. A. (1975). Medical complications of induced abortions. *Obstet. Gynecol. Survey*, **30**, 30–3

Rofe, A., Abramovici, H., David, A., Atad, J. and Lewin, A. (1980). Extraovular instillation of normal saline for termination of midtrimester pregnancy. *Int. J. Gynaecol. Obstet.*, **18**, 351–3

Shapiro, A. (1975). Extraovular prostaglandins $F_{2\alpha}$ for early midtrimester abortion. *Am. J. Obstet. Gynecol.*, **121**, 333–6

Schulman, H., Saldana, L., Tsai, T., Leibman, T., Cunningham, M. and Randolph, G. (1974). Prostaglandin E_2 induced abortion with vaginal suppositories in a contraceptive diaphragm. *Prostaglandins*, **7**, 195–205

Wiqvist, N., Bygdeman, M., Papageorgin, C. and Toppozada, M. K. (1974). Intrauterine administration of prostaglandins by extraamniotic route. *Prostaglandins*, **7**, 193–205

4
Stretch-induced Abortion at Mid-trimester

Y. MANABE, A. NAKAJIMA and Y. YOSHIDA

INTRODUCTION

Stretching of the uterus by various foreign bodies, such as laminaria, rubber bougie, catheter, and balloon causes significant cervical softening and onset of labor. At mid-trimester, the efficiency of these foreign bodies for inducing labor has not always been sufficient to achieve abortion without the use of oxytocis (Manabe, 1969). These foreign bodies had been used for labor induction at term, but were discontinued in many countries due to the risk of infection (Manabe *et al.*, 1982c). These techniques were also employed in mid-trimester abortion to replace the hypertonic saline method which proved to involve various risks. With the advances in prostaglandins (PG) research, the use of various foreign bodies at mid-trimester is on the decline even in Japan, with the exception of laminaria–balloon (Manabe and Nakajima, 1972a) and Rivanol–catheter method (Manabe, 1969; Ingemanson, 1979).

The mechanism of cervical softening and onset of labor by these methods is of physiological interest, since these phenomena occur even without oxytocics (Manabe *et al.*, 1973). Stretch-induced release of PG is involved in the mode of action of those foreign bodies (Manabe *et al.*, 1982c; in press).

CLINICAL APPLICATION

Laminaria–balloon method

Patients

Eighty patients between 13 and 22 weeks of gestation were divided into the early (Group I: 13–17 weeks, $n = 40$) and late (Group II: 18–22 weeks, $n = 40$) mid-trimester groups. Only subjects who had not experienced full-term delivery were selected.

Procedure

After dilatation with Hegar dilators, three to six laminaria were inserted into the cervix. Forty-eight hours later the laminaria were replaced with a 100-ml

31

capacity rubber balloon (Komine Rubber Co., Tokyo) (Fig. 4.1a), which was then inflated with 150 ml (Group I) and 180 ml (Group II) of water; traction of 600–800 g was given and oxytocin–$PGF_{2\alpha}$ drip-infusion was started usually at 9 a.m. The infusion speed was adjusted so that 500 ml of 5% glucose, containing 10 IU and 6 mg $PGF_{2\alpha}$, could be given in 12 h. When abortion did not occur within the first 12 h, drip-infusion and traction of balloon were stopped at 9 p.m. and resumed at 9 a.m. the next morning. Appropriate chemoprophylaxis was administered, and after fetal and placental delivery, all residual placenta was removed.

Results

Excluding the 48 h laminaria pretreatment, the abortion rates for Groups I and II were 70% (28/40) and 88% (35/40) respectively (Table 4.1). Abortion usually occurred during the drip-infusion and traction period, and in only four (10%) and two (2%) cases in Groups I and II, did abortion occur when these treatments were suspended. Abortion time was significantly shorter in Group II than in Group I.

The major side effects were nausea, vomiting and diarrhea due to the use of $PGF_{2\alpha}$ (Table 4.2). In one case approximately 100 ml of bleeding was noted upon laminaria insertion; this subject was excluded from the study since partial placenta praevia was suspected.

The longer the time of laminaria pretreatment (48 versus 24 h), the better the efficiency of cervical softening and dilatation, since the purpose of inserting the laminaria is cervical softening rather than dilatation.

Table 4.1 Abortion time and cumulative abortion rates (in parentheses) in the laminaria–balloon method supplemented by oxytocin plus $PGF_{2\alpha}$ drip infusion

Gestational week and no. of cases	Abortion time (h)[1] and cumulative abortion rates (%)			
	0–12[2]	*12–24*	*24–36*	*36–48*
13th to 17th (n = 40)	28 (70%)	2 (75%)	8 (95%)	2 (95%)
18th to 22nd (n = 40)	35 (88%)	2 (93%)	3 (100%)	0 (100%)

[1] Not including the 48 h laminaria pretreatment time
[2] Period of drip-infusion (oxytocin + $PGF_{2\alpha}$) and traction
   Data from Manabe and Manabe, 1981a, p. 85

Table 4.2 Side effects in mid-trimester abortion by laminaria–balloon, catheters, and catheter–balloon methods

	Laminaria–balloon (n = 80)	Catheters (n = 40)	Catheter–balloon (n = 40)
Nausea or vomiting	10 (13%)	9 (23%)	13 (33%)
Diarrhea	2 (3%)	2 (5%)	4 (10%)
Bleeding over 500 ml	0	0	0
Fever above 38°C	0	6 (15%)[1]	4 (10%)[1]

[1] Of the 10 cases (six plus four), the fever subsided in six within 24 h without additional chemotherapy

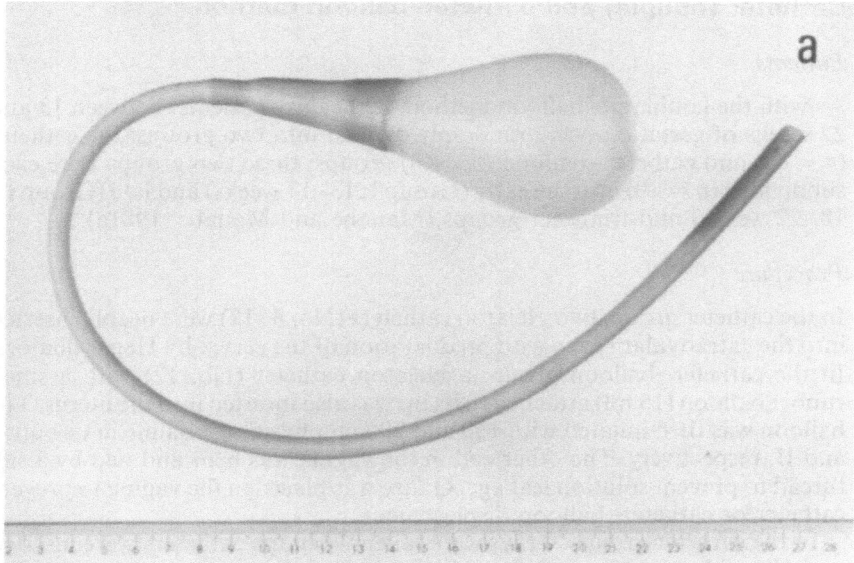

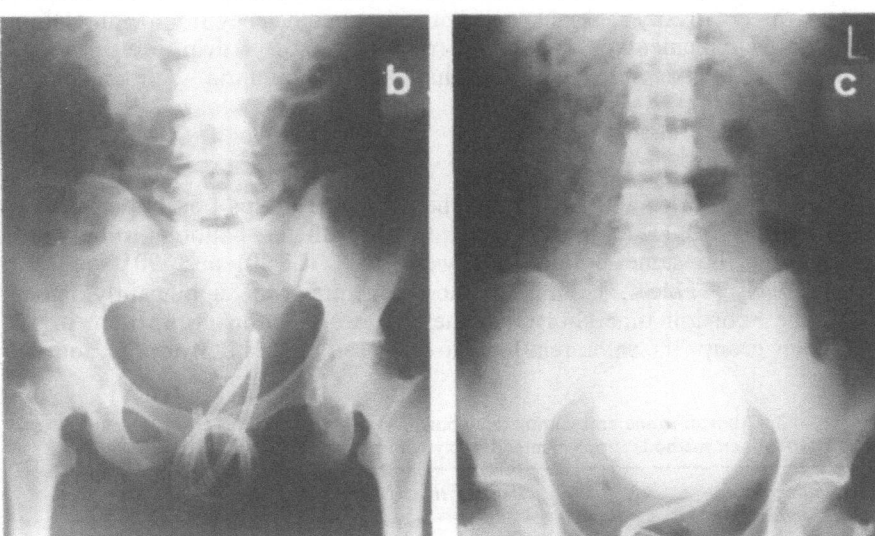

Fig. 4.1 (a) Rubber balloon used by the authors. When applied in the uterus, this device induces both cervical softening and uterine activity at mid-trimester and at term, and similar uterine activity at post-partum. Pattern of uterine contractions cannot be differentiated from those noted at spontaneous normal term delivery. Rubber thickness is an important factor; if it is too thin, a portion of it may come out due to traction. (b) Two Nelaton catheters (external diameter 9 mm) were completely inserted beyond the internal cervical os for uterine streching. Note the proper curling of catheters in the lower uterine region (22nd week of pregnancy) (Manabe *et al.*, 1981b, p. 63). (c) Intrauterine position of a balloon–catheter applied for uterine stretching (20th week of pregnancy) (Manabe and Manabe, 1981a, p. 85)

Catheter (bougie) and catheter–balloon method

Patients

As with the laminaria–balloon method, 80 healthy patients, between 13 and 22 weeks of gestation, were randomly divided into two groups: the catheter ($n = 40$) and catheter–balloon ($n = 40$) groups; these two groups were each subdivided ($n = 20$) into the early (Group I: 13–17 weeks) and late (Group II: 18–22 weeks) mid-trimester groups (Manabe and Manabe, 1981a).

Procedure

In the catheter group, two Nelaton catheters (No. 8–12) were deeply inserted into the extraovular space with predilatation of the cervix by Hegar dilators. In the catheter–balloon group, a Nelaton catheter (No. 12) with a small rubber balloon (15 ml) attached to its tip was also inserted into the uterus. The balloon was then inflated with 150 and 200 ml physiologic saline in Groups I and II, respectively. The other end in the vagina was bent and tied by a silk thread to prevent solution leakage. Gauze was placed in the vagina to prevent catheter or catheter–balloon displacement.

In the catheter group, X-rays were taken when the catheters were inserted and when labor became significant to determine any changes in the position of the catheters or any regional specificities in the efficiency for starting labor.

Daily supplementary treatment (oxytocin–$PGF_{2\alpha}$ drip infusion) and chemoprophylaxis were identical to that with the laminaria–balloon method (12 h duration).

Results

The abortion rates within 72 h for the catheter Groups I and II were 60% (12/20) and 75% (15/20), respectively; for the catheter–balloon Groups I and II during the same period they were 75% (15/20) and 90% (18/20), respectively (Table 4.3). Thus, the abortion rates were significantly higher, and the abortion time shorter in the catheter–balloon group than in the catheter group; the same relationship was seen between Groups II and I.

Table 4.3 Abortion time and cumulative abortion rates (in parentheses) in the catheter and catheter-balloon methods supplemented by oxytocin plus $PGF_{2\alpha}$ drip infusion.)

Gestational week and no. of cases	*Abortion time* (h) *and cumulative abortion rates* (%)			
	0–24	*24–48*	*48–72*	*Over 72*
13th to 17th ($n = 40$)				
Catheter ($n = 40$)	0	3 (15%)	9 (60%)	8 (100%)
Catheter–balloon ($n = 20$)	2 (10%)	8 (50%)	5 (75%)	5 (100%)
18th to 22nd ($n = 40$)				
Catheter ($n = 20$)	1 (5%)	4 (25%)	10 (75%)	5 (100%)
Catheter–balloon ($n = 20$)	3 (15%)	8 (55%)	7 (90%)	2 (100%)

Data from Manabe and Manabe, 1981a, p. 85

Figures 4.1b and 4.1c show the intrauterine position of the catheters and catheter–balloon in one representative case with each respective method. Figure 4.2 illustrates the position of the Nelaton catheter in the extraovular space when inserted in 10 randomly selected cases. When labor became significant, X-ray photographs usually showed the catheters in different positions from those in the initial stage of the operation.

As shown in Table 4.2, nausea and diarrhea were noted in 22 (28 %) and six (8 %) cases in the respective methods. Upon insertion of the catheter, fresh bleeding was noted in some cases, probably because the catheter hits the placenta; the bleeding stopped soon after finding a resistance-free region or cutting the superfluous part of the catheters. The amount of post-partum bleeding was small because of the immediate examination of the residual placenta.

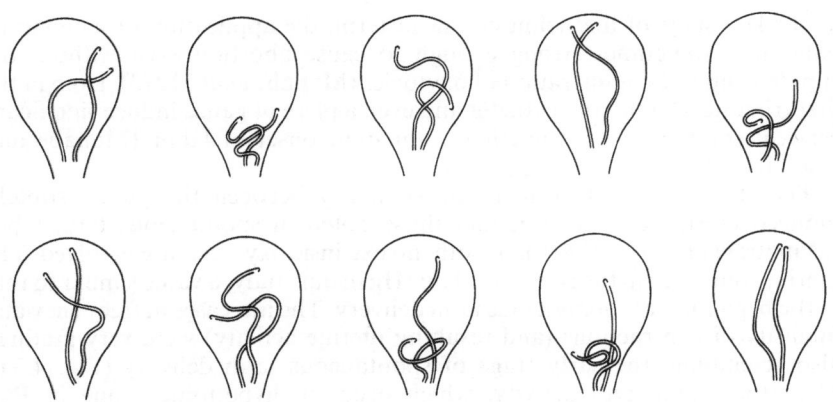

Fig. 4.2 The position of two catheters in the extraovular space in 10 randomly selected cases in whom artificial abortion at mid-trimester was attempted by uterine stretching. Arbitrary sites of catheters are characteristic, thus stimulating unspecified regions of the uterus (Manabe and Manabe, 1981a, p. 85)

Comments on stretch-induced abortion

The laminaria–balloon method is now commonly used in Japan and may be competitive with other current techniques which use PG only, when the laminaria pretreatment time is not included in the abortion time. Using this method, 469 cases were studied (Yanagita *et al.*, 1971), and the abortion time and cumulative abortion rates were essentially similar to our results; fever above 38 °C was seen in only six out of the total cases (1.3 %). Thus, the risk of endometritis with this method was negligible, because of chemoprophylaxis and reduced abortion time from the use of oxytocics.

Using the catheter or catheter–balloon method, the rate of endometritis was relatively higher than that with the laminaria–balloon method (Manabe, 1969; Manabe and Manabe, 1981a). Favorable results were reported in 88 mid-trimester abortions using a Foley catheter with an inflated 75-ml balloon and oxytocin (Godsick, 1971).

The laminaria−balloon or Rivanol−catheter method is apparently superior to either the catheter or catheter−balloon method. Mid-trimester abortion by the Rivanol−catheter results from the mutual and combined action of the catheter and solution; namely, uterine stretching by a liquid and a solid foreign body (Manabe, 1969). With this method the importance of the Nelaton or Foley catheter with its balloon expanded has been discussed in relation to the abortion time (Ingemanson, 1979).

THEORETICAL DISCUSSION

Characteristics of uterine activity

In the late stage of mid-trimester, as at term, the application of laminaria− balloon is sometimes strong enough to cause abortion even without the supplementary administration of oxytocics (Manabe et al., 1973). Even in the first trimester, laminaria, catheter and even a piece of gauze induce significant cervical softening and, sometimes, apparent onset of labor (Manabe and Manabe, 1981b).

The characteristic feature is the similarity between the purely stretch-induced uterine contractions and those noted in spontaneous term labor (Manabe et al., 1973, 1981b): in both, no extrinsic oxytocics are involved. The uterine tonus was in the range of 10 mmHg in our study, a value similar to that at the beginning of spontaneous term delivery. The increases in frequency and intensity of contractions (and resulting uterine activity) were very gradual, also resembling the early stage of spontaneous term delivery (Fig. 4.3a). Hypertonia and hyperactivity, which occur in hypertonic saline or PG-induced abortion (Lauersen et al., 1974), were never observed.

Steroid hormones

Plasma estrogens and progesterone levels before and during normal delivery did not change (Okada et al., 1974); likewise, the plasma levels of these hormones were not significantly altered during the mid-trimester abortion either by the laminaria−balloon or by rubber bougie method (Manabe, 1970; Manabe et al., 1981a).

Histology of amnion and chorion

In placenta delivered by uterine stretching, normal histological integrity and viability, as confirmed by light and electron microscopy (Manabe and Yoshida, 1973), and autoradiography (Manabe et al., 1981b), are in accord with the unchanged hormonal levels in blood (Figs 4.4 and 4.5). These findings, together with the fact that the fetus is usually delivered unharmed (alive) when it is large enough to withstand the mechanics of labor, suggest

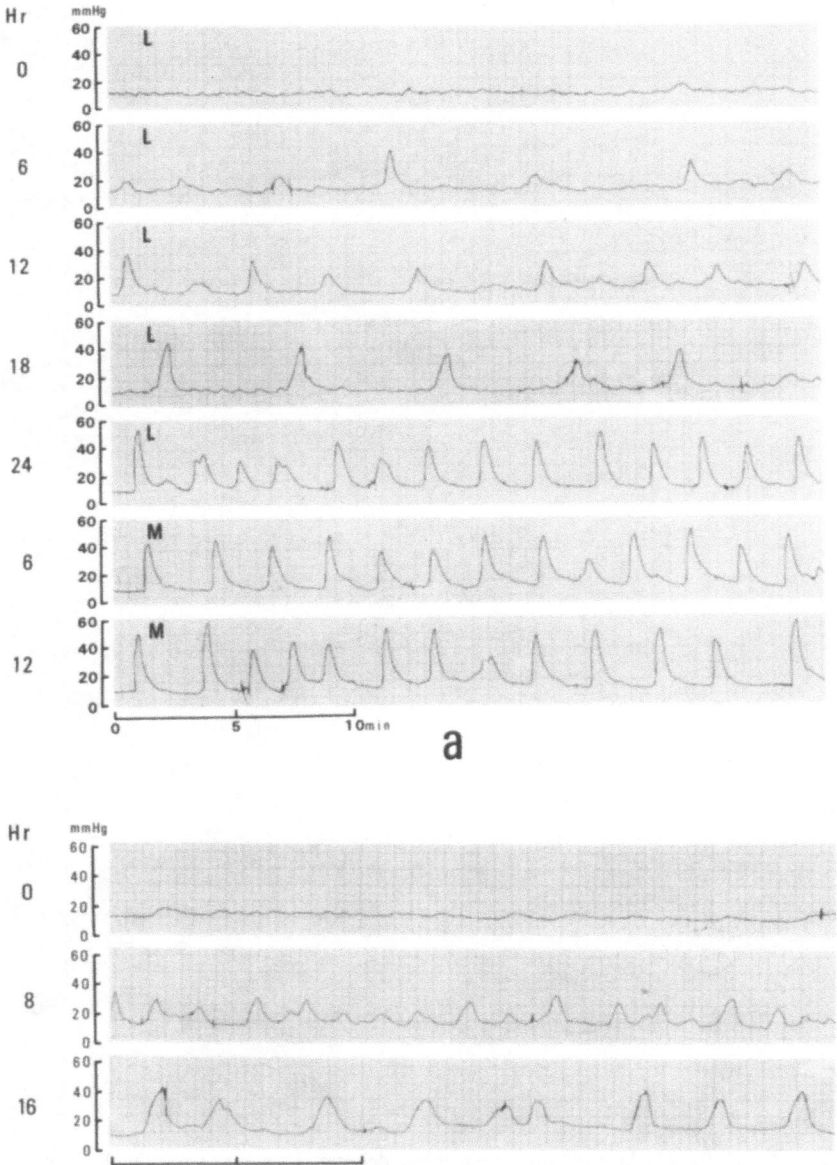

Fig. 4.3 **(a)** Development of uterine activity during laminaria–balloon treatment (20th week of pregnancy). Hours after laminaria (L) and balloon (M) insertion are listed at the left. In this case, the laminaria was replaced with the balloon after 24 h (Manabe *et al.*, 1973, p. 753). **(b)** Evolution of uterine activity during uterine stretching under continuous extradural and caudal blocks (22nd week of pregnancy) (Manabe *et al.*, 1981b, p. 63)

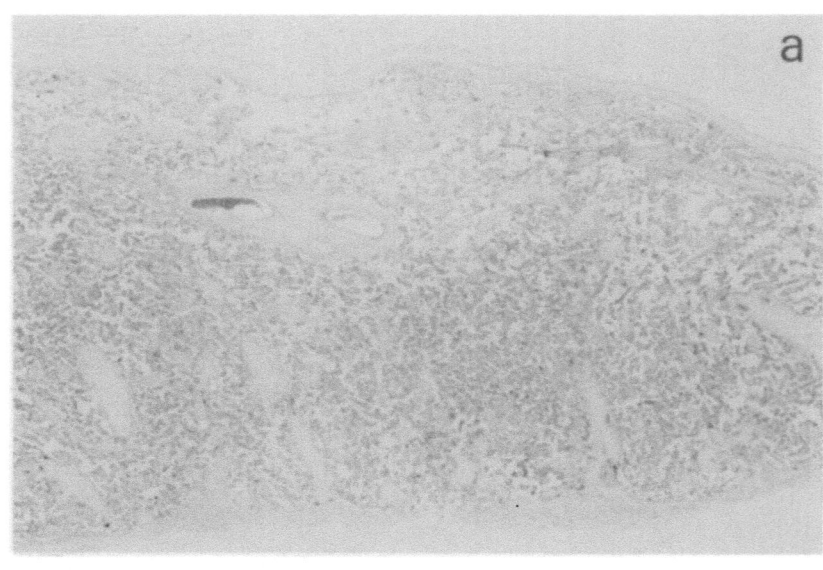

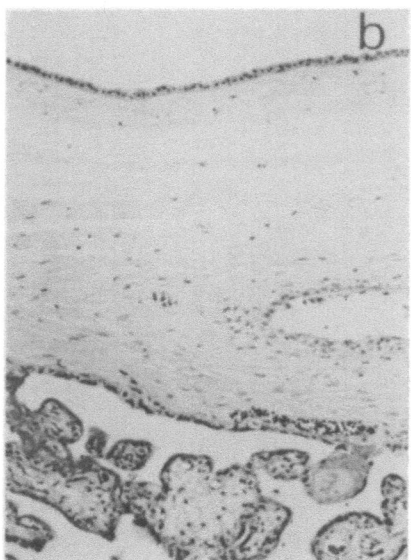
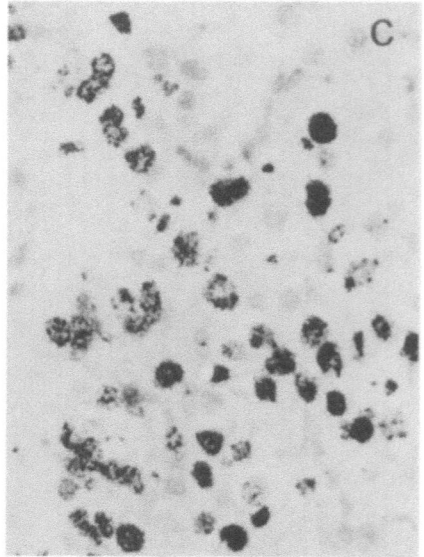

Fig. 4.4 (a) Full-thickness section of a placenta delivered by uterine stretching by laminaria–balloon method (21st week of pregnancy). The fetus was delivered alive. Histological normality of the entire thickness of the plancenta is maintained. Fetal side upward, maternal side downward (H & E × 2.5) (Manabe and Yoshida, 1973, p. 379, 61). (b) Details from the placenta illustrated in Fig. 4.4a. Normal histological features of the amnion and the underlying chorion are preserved. No inflammatory cell infiltration is observed (H & E × 55) (Manabe and Yoshida, 1973, p. 379). (c) Autoradiograph of the chorion of the placenta delivered by uterine stretching by catheters method (22nd week of pregnancy). The fetus was delivered alive. Note the intensely labeled cytotrophoblastic cells (H & E × 210) (Manabe *et al.*, 1981b, p. 63)

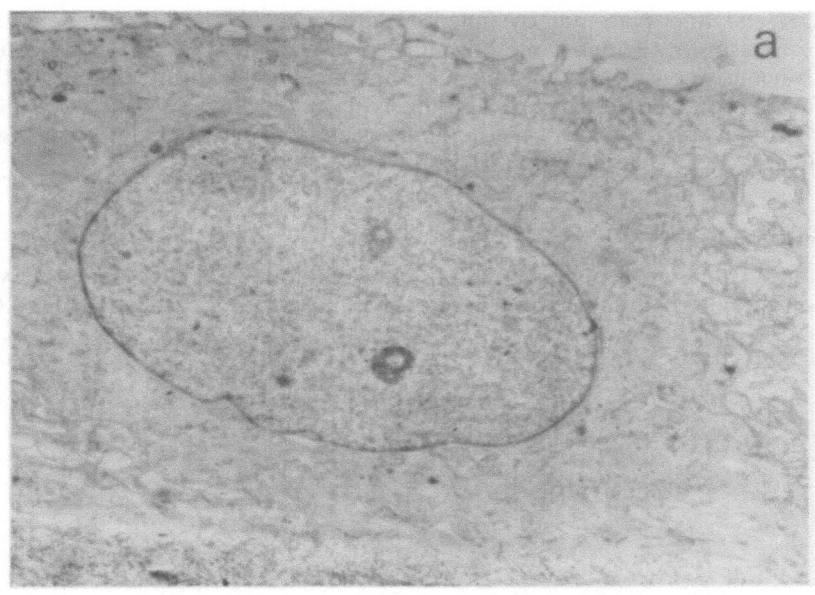

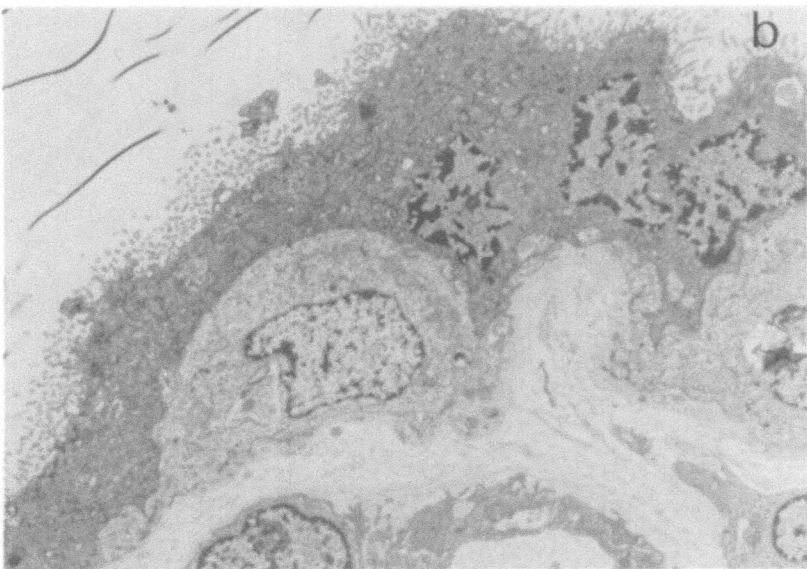

Fig. 4.5 (a) Electron micrograph of an amniotic epithelial cell (clear cell type) and underlying fibrous layer of the placenta shown in Fig. 4.4a. Normality of cellular elements is maintained ($\times 8400$) (Manabe and Yoshida, 1973, p. 379). (b) Electron micrograph of the chorion from the placenta shown in Fig. 4.4a. Syncytiotrophoblast and cytotrophoblast are normal. The trophoblastic basement membrane and fetal capillary are intact. Neither pyknotic nuclei nor cytoplasmic vacuoles are seen. Numerous cell organelles show normal integrity; no sign of cell degeneration ($\times 4370$)

that fetal and placental dysfunctions are probably not involved in the mechanisms of the onset of labor induced by uterine stretching. It was once erroneously considered that functional and histological disintegrations of the placenta could be the cause of labor by hypertonic saline. This misconception is certainly attributable to the random selection of experimental parameters which lacked scientific basis (Manabe and Nakajima, 1972).

Oxytocin and spinal reflex mechanisms

In mid-trimester, complete epidural and caudal block of the afferent nerves from the uterus was performed before the insertion of catheters (Fig. 4.6),

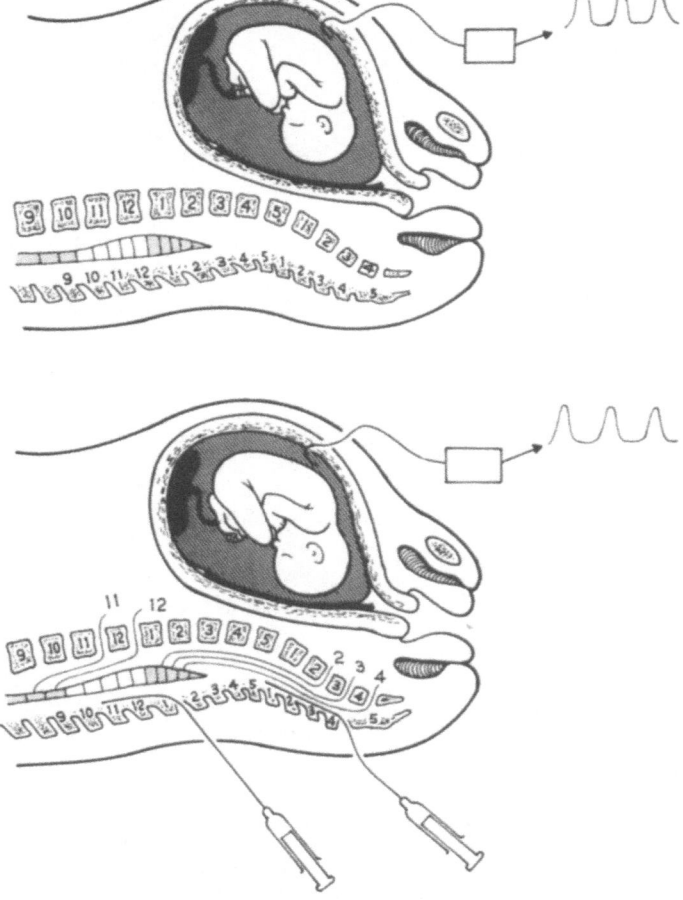

Fig. 4.6 Schematic representation of intrauterine application of Nelaton catheter (top), the same device with continuous extradural and caudal blocks (bottom), and the method for recording intrauterine pressure. See text for details (Manabe *et al.*, 1981b, p. 63)

laminaria or a balloon into the uterus, and this nerve block was maintained throughout the study. Uterine activity showed no significant difference between the nerve block and non-nerve block groups (Fig. 4.3b) (Manabe *et al.*, 1981b, 1982d). Similar results were reported in mid-trimester abortion by laminaria and balloon in a patient with a complete spinal block below the level of T5 (Nakajima and Hayashi, 1965).

Plasma oxytocin values did not increase significantly in either the normal or the nerve block patients in stretch-induced labor at mid-trimester (Manabe *et al.*, 1982). Moreover, intrinsic oxytocin did not participate in balloon-induced labor at term (Fisch *et al.*, 1964). The failure to detect oxytocin in the plasma during mid-trimester agrees with similar findings in the second stage of labor at term (Chard *et al.*, 1970).

Stretch-induced release of PG

When mechanical uterine stretching was applied to term patients not in labor, significant cervical softening, and the onset and progress of labor, was achieved (Manabe *et al.*, 1982a,c, 1984). Stretching of the myometrium results in the release of PG (Poyser *et al.*, 1971; Kloeck and Jung, 1973). Exogenous PG are capable of inducing cervical softening and labor. Serial analyses of PGE and/or PGF in amniotic fluid during delivery induced by rubber bougie or balloon, revealed the rise of these PG values with the progress of cervical softening and labor (Table 4.4) (Manabe *et al.*, 1982c, 1984). Similar results were obtained in purely stretch-induced labor at mid-trimester (unpublished data). Significant onset of labor always preceded the significant rise of the levels of PG. There is no evidence that increased PG production precedes urea-induced uterine contractions (Dubin *et al.*, 1977). Thus, increased release of PG is not the trigger of labor but a result of uterine distension and/or

Table 4.4 Levels of PGE and PGF (pg/ml) in amniotic fluid during cervical softening and labor at term induced by uterine stretching by rubber bougies

Case no.	cervical dilatation (cm)							
	2 (before stretch)		3–4		5–6		9–10	
	PGE	PGF	PGE	PGF	PGE	PGF	PGE	PGF
1	84	91	698	764	2230	943	1695	4251
2	565	124	1108	281	996	1918	3350	3612
3	325	52	311	94	788	487	812	967
4	752	528	498	680	882	1724	1326	2017
5	571	253	783	1178	408	3150	3047	2980
6	196	365	1512	838	1983	512	2305	786
7	362	865	1115	1736	4208	2068	4924	6275
Mean	408	324	864	796	1142	1543	2494	2984
SE	88	111	156	207	495	364	530	735

Data from Manabe *et al.*, 1984

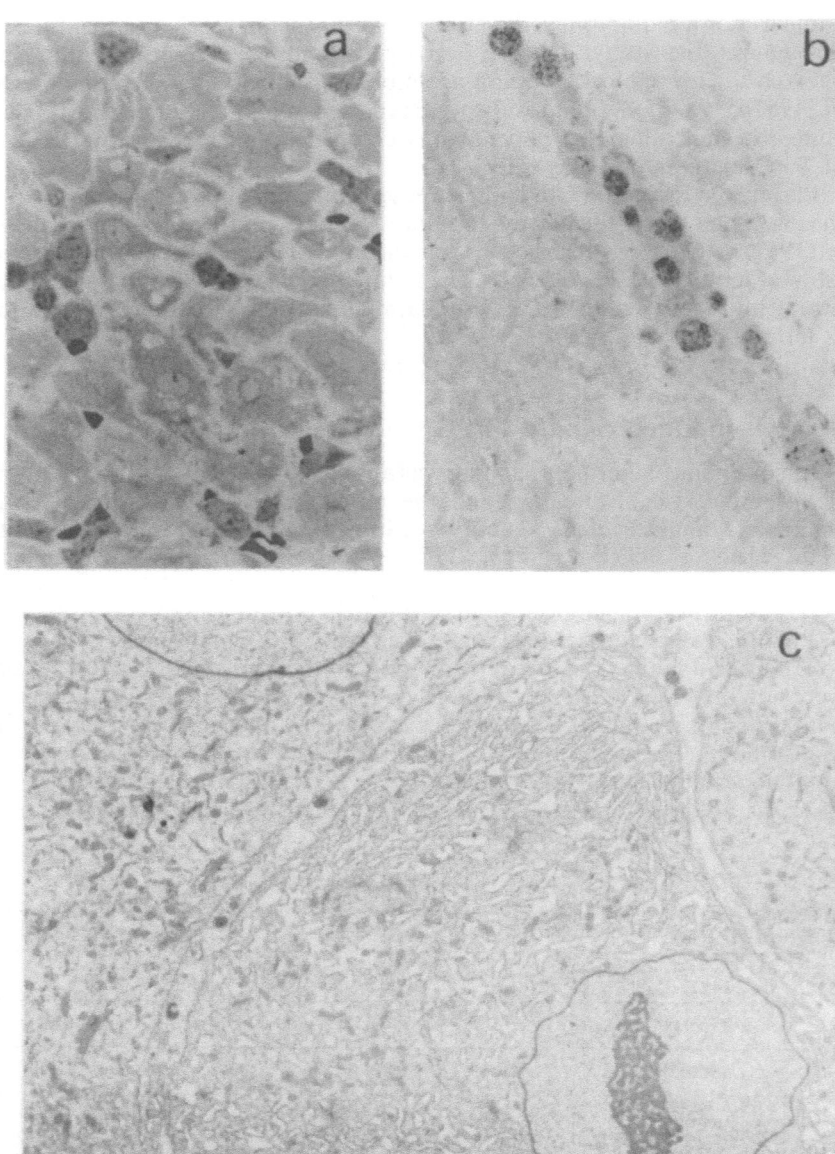

Fig. 4.7 (a) Decidual cells in the compact layer of decidua parietalis, obtained from a woman (15th week of pregnancy) when purely stretch-induced uterine activity was regular and strong using the laminaria–balloon method. Entirely normal cell characteristics are preserved. The cells do not show any degeneration such as vacuolization of the cytoplasm, nor pyknotic, vacuolated, or disintegrated nuclei. Many white spots show fat droplets; not vacuolization. Note many protrusions radiating from the rim of the cells which contain numerous fine secretory granules (Yoshide *et al.*, 1980). These findings are more clearly visible in an electron micrograph shown

subsequently induced labor (Salmon and Amy, 1973; Manabe *et al.*, 1982c, 1984).

During mid-trimester or at term, uterine stretching by various solutions, such as 0.1 % Rivanol, glucose, physiological saline, and distilled water, are also capable of inducing cervical softening and labor (Manabe, 1972). The rise of PG values in amniotic fluid was reported during Rivanol–catheter or hypertonic solution-induced abortion (Dubin *et al.*, 1977; Ölund *et al.*, 1980). When applied in the uterus, hypertonic solutions probably cause a continuous influx of body fluid into the uterus until equilibrium between intra- and extrauterine osmolarity is attained. These solutions, similar to solid foreign bodies, may exert a stretching effect to the uterus resulting in the release of PG (Manabe *et al.*, 1982c).

During the progress of pregnancy the cervix gradually softens towards term. The PG values in amniotic fluid increase gradually as term approaches (Salmon and Amy, 1973). Even the growing conceptus and increasing amniotic fluid would physiologically stretch the myometrium; this could result in cervical softening and elevation of uterine contractility as gestation progresses, thereby releasing PG.

Mathematical analysis of the stretch effect to the lower uterine segment and cervix by the fetal head has been performed; after artificial or spontaneous rupture of the membranes the fetal head comes into direct contact with the uterus, and the physical force applied by the head to the contacting regions of the uterus increases (Yasui, 1974), thus releasing PG (unpublished data).

Sources and mechanisms of PG synthesis

Because a high concentration of PG has been found in extracts of decidua it was postulated that PG are mainly formed in decidual cells and are related to the onset of labor (Karim and Devlin, 1967). The total amount of myometrium at term (600–700 g), which generates and releases PG by its direct distension and/or contractions, is considerably larger than that of decidua which significantly and relatively decreases towards term. The major source of the synthesis and release of PG is probably the myometrium and not the decidua both during stretch-induced abortion at mid-trimester and during normal term delivery (Manabe *et al.*, in press), though the decidua and fetal membranes certainly take part in the generation and release of PG to some extent (Keirse, 1978).

Decidual degeneration may lead to the leakage of phospholipase A_2 from

---

in Fig. 4.7c. Section was prepared from Epon embedding in 1 μm thickness (H & E × 504). (b) Cytochemical demonstration of acid phosphatase in decidual cells as in Fig. 4.7a. Numerous secretory granules in the many protrusions radiating from the cytoplasmic rim show strong acid phosphatase activity. Reaction products (precipitations) in the secretory granules and Golgi membranes reveal the sites of acid phosphatase activity (× 92 400). (c) Electron micrograph of decidual cells in the compact layer obtained from the woman as in Fig. 4.7a. Neither pyknotic nuclei nor cytoplasmic vacuoles are seen. Numerous cell organelles show normal integrity; no sign of cell degeneration. Some secretory granules around the cell are visible (× 4200) the lysosomes, and the resulting formation of PG precursors from phospholipids could be the cause of onset of labor induced by saline (Gustavii, 1974). In an attempt to study this possibility, decidua parietalis was obtained either when significant labor was established or abortion was achieved in various stretch-induced abortions including those using the Rivanol–catheter method. Neither such degenerative changes nor leakage into the cell cytoplasm of lysosomal 'marker' enzyme acid phosphatase has been found (Fig. 4.7), i.e. the same findings as the control before the treatment. Furthermore, basal decidua which was obtained after spontaneous or stretch-induced delivery at term also showed the same cell integrity, excepting some partial physiological necrotic changes known at term (McCombs and Craig, 1964); this could not be differentiated from the control obtained by Cesarean section (unpublished data).

The importance of lysosomal enzymes in the control of uterine PG production has also been questioned biochemically (Batra and Bengtsson, 1976). The decidual degeneration, which Gustavii (1974) observed, could be a secondary event resulting either from the detachment of the fetal membranes from the uterus by solution, or from strong uterine contractions which were already initiated by uterine distension; the decidual degeneration, when it occurs, could probably be excluded as the cause of onset of labor.

IUDs in rats release PG, and the administration of indomethacin inhibits such a release (Chaudhuri, 1973). Even in post-menopausal patients, significant cervical softening was brought about by catheter application, probably due to the involvement of PG (Manabe et al., 1982b). By means of a rubber balloon, onset of regular and strong uterine contractions, which were suppressed by indomethacin, was noted in post-partum patients where, of course, neither decidua nor fetal membranes are involved; the contraction patterns (tonus, intensity and frequency of contractions) could not be differentiated from those noted in either stretch-induced mid-trimester, or spontaneous or stretch-induced term delivery (unpublished data). Therefore, PG of decidual and placental origins are probably neither motivator of labor nor the major source of PG release during labor.

As both uterine stretching and/or the resulting contractions seem to cause the release of PG, its total release could be a combination of these two factors (Manabe et al., 1982c). Hypothetically, uterine distension and/or the resulting contractions may cause the following sequence of events: myometrial ischemia (Bülbring, 1953), progressive increase in mitochondrial free fatty acids (Lindenmayer et al., 1968; Boime et al., 1970; McGiff et al., 1970), and finally the release of PG. The latter part of this hypothesis has also been proposed (Batra and Bengtsson, 1976).

PG do not appear to be stored in significant amounts in tissues, but are instead released as a result of de novo biosynthesis by various stimuli (Piper and Vane, 1971). Many organs have been demonstrated to have an ability to release PG when subjected to mechanical stretch. The release of a PG-like substance was demonstrated upon distension of the stomach (Bennett et al., 1967), bladder (Gilmore, 1971), and lungs (Berry et al., 1971). Thus, any organ, including the myometrium, seems capable of releasing PG upon mechanical stimulation.

Myogenic activity of the uterus

Intracellular (Goto and Woodbury, 1958; Nakajima and Tauchi, 1970) and extracellular (Nakajima and Tauchi, 1970; Manabe and Nakajima, 1971) electrode studies indicated that onset of myometrial activities always immediately follows distension (Fig. 4.8a,b). Moderate stretching of most

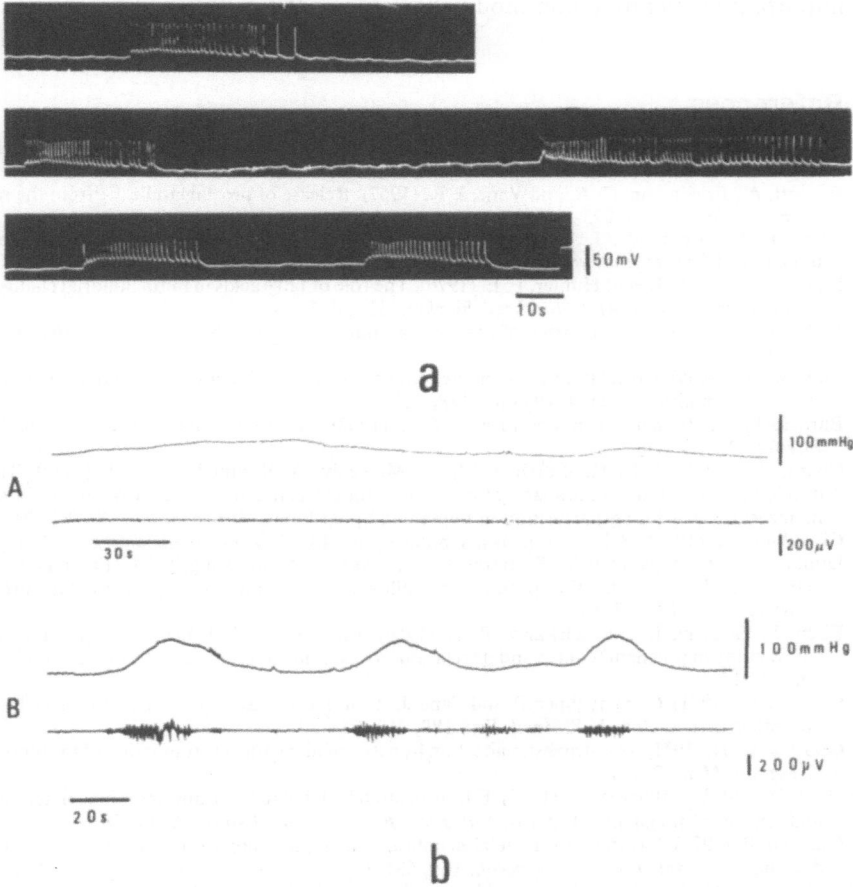

Fig. 4.8 (a) Effect of stretch on membrane and action potentials, and rate of spike discharge in uterine muscle of a rat at the late stage of pregnancy. Upper tracing: *in situ* length; middle tracing: a muscle was stretched to about twice its *in situ* length. Note the increase in spike frequency and the fall of membrane potential; Lower tracing: a muscle was extended three times its *in situ* length. Further depolarization of the membrane potenial and the rise of the rate of spike discharge are observed (Nakajima and Tauchi, 1970, p. 692). (b) Uterine activity induced by mechanical stretching of the lower uterine segment and cervix by rubber balloon in a normal term subject; simultaneous recording of intra-amniotic pressure (upper tracing) and electromyogram (lower tracing). Electrode was placed 7 cm above the external cervical os. **A:** Immediately after stretch application. Almost no mechanical and electrical activities are seen. **B:** 90 min after stretching. Note apparent inauguration of mechanical and electrical activities. This study demonstrates the stretch dependency of uterine activity (Nakajima and Tauchi, 1970, p. 692)

smooth muscles causes the depolarization, initiation of spiking, or an increase in spike frequency, and therefore an increase in tension and oxygen consumption (Bülbring, 1955; Burnstock *et al.*, 1963). This attribute of the uterus, as a smooth muscle, could be the real triggering and promoting factor in stretch-induced and spontaneous uterine activity both at mid-trimester and at term, although a similar stretch-dependent release of PG plays some important accelerating and modulating role in the progress of labor.

References

Batra, S. and Bengtsson, L. P. (1976). Mechanism for increased production of prostaglandins in labour. *Lancet*, 1, 1164–5

Bennett, A., Friedmann, C. A. and Vane, J. R. (1967). Release of prostaglandin E$_1$ from the rat stomach. *Nature*, 216, 873–6

Berry, E. M., Edmonds, J. F. and Wyllie, J. H. (1971). Release of prostaglandin E$_2$ and unidentified factors from ventilated lungs. *Br. J. Surg.*, 58, 189–98

Boime, I., Smith, E. E. and Hunter, F. E. (1970). The role of fatty acids in mitochondrial changes during liver ischemia, *Arch. Biochem. Biophys.*, 139, 425–43

Bülbring, E. (1953). Measurements of oxygen consumption in smooth muscle. *J. Physiol.*, 122, 111–34

Bülbring, E. (1955). Correlation between membrane potential, spike discharge and tension and tension in smooth muscle. *J. Physiol.*, 128, 200–21

Burnstock, G., Holman, M. E. and Prosser, C. L. (1963). Electrophysiology of smooth muscle. *Physiol. Rev.*, 43, 482–527

Chard, T., Boyd, N. R. H., Forsling, M. L., McNeilly, A. S. and Landon, J. (1970). The development of a radioimmunoassay for oxytocin: the extraction of oxytocin from plasma, and its measurement during parturition in human and goat blood. *J. Endocrinol.*, 48, 223–34

Chaudhuri, G. (1973). Release of prostaglandins by the I.U.C.D. *Prostaglandins*, 3, 773–84

Dubin, N. H., Ghodgaonkar, R. B., Baros, N. A., Blake, D. A. and King, T. M. (1977). Uterine activity and prostaglandin production following intraamniotic hyperosmolar urea. *Prostaglandins*, 14, 753–62

Fisch, L., Sala, N. L. and Schwarcz, R. L. (1964). Effect of cervical dilatation upon uterine contractility in pregnant women and its relation to oxytocin secretion. *Am. J. Obstet. Gynecol.*, 90, 108–14

Gilmore, M. (1971). Cited by Piper, P. and Vane, J. R. In: The release of prostaglandins from lung and other tissues. *Ann. N.Y. Acad. Sci.*, 180, 363–85

Godsick, W. H. (1971). Mid-trimester abortion by extra-ovular catheter stimulation of the uterus. *J. Reprod. Med.*, 7, 281

Goto, M. and Woodbury, J. W. (1958). Effects of stretch and NaCl on transmembrane potentials and tension of pregnant rat uterus. *Fed. Proc. Fed. Am. Soc. Exp. Biol.*, 17, 58

Gustavii, B. (1974). Sweeping of the fetal membranes by a physiologic saline solution: effect on decidual cells. *Am. J. Obstet. Gynecol.*, 120, 531–6

Ingemanson, C.-A. (1979). The ethacridine–catheter method in second-trimester abortion. In Zatuchi, Sciarra, and Speidel, (eds.) *Pregnancy Termination, Procedures, Safety and New Developments.* pp. 282–9. (Hagerstown: Harper & Row)

Karim, S. M. M. and Devlin, J. (1967). Prostaglandin content of amniotic fluid during pregnancy and labour. *J. Obstet. Gynaecol. Br. Commonw.*, 74, 230–4

Keirse, M. J. N. C. (1978). Biosynthesis and metabolism of prostaglandins in the pregnant human uterus. *Adv. Prostaglandin Thromboxane Res.*, 4, 78–102

Kloeck, F. K. and Jung, H. (1973). In vitro release of prostaglandins from the human myometrium under the influence of stretching. *Am. J. Obstet. Gynecol.*, 115, 1066–9

Lauersen, N. H., Wilson, K. H., Beling, C. G. and Fuchs, R. (1974). Comparison of prostaglandin F$_{2\alpha}$ and hypertonic saline for induction of mid-trimester abortion. *Am. J. Obstet. Gynecol.*, 120, 875–89

Lindenmayer, G. E., Sordahl, L. A. and Schwartz, A. (1968). Reevaluation of oxidative phosphorylation in cardiac mitochondria from normal animals and animals in heart failure. *Circulation Rec.*, **23**, 439–450

Manabe, Y. (1969). Artificial abortion in midpregnancy by mechanical stimulation of the uterus. *Am. J. Obstet. Gynecol.*, **105**, 132–46

Manabe, Y. (1970). Plasma progesterine levels during bougie-induced abortion at mid-pregnancy. *J. Endocrinol.*, **46**, 127–8

Manabe, Y. (1972). Interruption of pregnancy at midterm by intrauterine application of solutions. *Obstet. Gynecol. Survey*, **27**, 701–10

Manabe, Y. and Manabe, A. (1981a). Abortion at midpregnancy by catheter or catheter–balloon supplemented by intravenous oxytocin and $PGF_{2\alpha}$. *Biol. Res. Pregnancy*, **2**, 85–9

Manabe, Y and Manabe, A. (1981b). Nelaton catheter versus laminaria for a safe and gradual cervical dilatation. *Contraception*, **24**, 53–60

Manabe, Y. and Nakajima, A. (1971). Changes of electrical activities by mechanical stimulation of the myometrium (Abstract). *Prog. Obstet. Gynecol.*, **23**, 358 (in Japanese)

Manabe, Y. and Nakajima, A. (1972a). Laminaria-metreurynter method of midterm abortion in Japan. *Obstet. Gynecol.*, **40**, 612–15

Manabe, Y. and Nakajima, A. (1972b). Divergence of opinion on placental damage due to hypertonic saline-induced abortion. *Am. J. Obstet. Gynecol.*, **114**, 1107–8

Manabe, Y. and Yoshida, Y. (1973). Light and electron microscopic studies of the placenta delivered by laminaria-metreurynter induced abortion at mid-pregnancy. *Endokronologie*, **61**, 379–84

Manabe, Y., Manabe, A. and Aso, (1981a). Plasma concentrations of oestrone, oestradiol, oestriol and progesterone during mechanical stretch-induced abortion at mid-trimester. *J. Endocrinol.*, 385–9

Manabe, Y., Manabe, A. and Sagawa, N. (1982a). Stretch-induced cervical softening and initiation of labor at term: a possible correlation with prostaglandins. *Acta Obstet. Gynecol. Scand.*, **61**, 279–80

Manabe, Y., Manabe, A. and Sakaguchi, M. (1982b). Nelaton catheter in non-gravidas for a safe and gradual cervical softening and dilatation: a possible involvement of prostaglandins. *Contraception*, **25**, 211–18

Manabe, Y., Manabe, A. and Takahashi, A. (1982c). F prostaglandin levels in amniotic fluid during balloon-induced cervical softening and labor at term. *Prostaglandins*, **23**, 247–56

Manabe, Y., Nakajima, A. and Griggs, J. F. (1973). Uterine contractility and placental histology in abortion by laminaria and metreurynter. *Obstet. Gynecol.*, **41**, 753–9

Manabe, Y., Okazaki, T. and Takahashi, A. (1984). Prostaglandins E and F in aminotic fluid during stretch-induced cervical softening and labor at term. *Gynecol. Obstet. Invest.* (In press)

Manabe, Y., Sagawa, N. and Takahashi, A. (1982d). Effect of continuous nerve block of the uterus on stretch-induced uterine activity in the mid-trimester. *J. Obstet. Gynaecol.*, **3**, 24–6

Manabe, Y., Sakaguchi, M. and Nakajima, A. (1981b). Initiation of uterine contractions by purely mechanical stretching of the uterus at midpregnancy. *Biol. Res. Pregnancy*, **2**, 63–9

McCombs, H. L. and Craig, J. M. (1964). Decidual necrosis in normal pregnancy. *Obstet. Gynecol.*, **24**, 436–42

McGiff, J. C., Crowshaw, K., Terragno, N. A., Lonigro, A. J., Strand, J. C., Williamson, M. A., Lee, J. B. and Ng, K. K. F. (1970). Prostaglandin-like substances appearing in canine renal venous blood during renal ischemia. *Circulation Res.*, **27**, 765–82

Nakajima, A. and Hayashi, T. (1965). Mechanism of onset of labor in a mid-trimester patient with complete spinal paralysis. *Sanka-To-Fujinka*, **32**, 1598–1601 (in Japanese)

Nakajima, A. and Tauchi, K. (1970). Lower uterine segment and induction of labor. *Sanfujinka-No-Jissai*, **19**, 692–701 (in Japanese)

Okada, D. M., Tulchinsky, D., Ross, J. W. and Hobel, C. J. (1974). Plasma estrone, estradiol, estriol, progesterone and cortisol in normal labor. *Am. J. Obstet. Gynecol.*, **119**, 502–7

Ölund, A. R., Kindahl, H., Oliw, E., Lindgren, J. A. and Larsson, B. (1980). Prostaglandins and thromboxanes in amniotic fluid during rivanol induced abortion and labour. *Prostaglandins*, **19**, 791–803

Piper, P. and Vane, J. R. (1971). The release of prostaglandins from lung and other tissues. *Ann. N. Y. Acad. Sci.*, **180**, 363–85

Poyser, N. L., Horton, E. W., Thompson, C. J. and Los, M. (1971). Identification of prostaglandin $F_{2\alpha}$ released by distention of guinea pig uterus in vitro. *Nature*, **230**, 526–8

Salmon, J. A. and Amy, J. J. (1973). Levels of prostaglandin $F_{2\alpha}$ in amniotic fluid during pregnancy and labour. *Prostaglandins,* **4,** 523–33

Yanagita, Y., Yoshida, Y. and Tanaka, F. (1971). Report on middle and late stage abortion in 469 American patients using laminaria sticks and balloons. *Excerpta Medica,* No. 234, 7th World Congress on Fertility and Sterility, Tokyo and Kyoto, p. 67

Yasui, S. (1974) Induction of labor and artifical rupture of the membranes. *Sanka-To-Fujinka,* **41,** 887–98 (in Japanese)

Yoshida, Y., Suzuki, H., Oshima, M. and Kasai, K. (1980). Development and secretory function of human decidual cells (2) Acid- phosphatase activity of secretory granules. *J. Clin. Electron Microsc.,* **13,** 402–3

5

Treatment of intrauterine fetal death by intracervical and extra-amniotic PGF$_{2\alpha}$/PGE$_2$

W. RATH, W. KUHN and H. KÜHNLE

Prior to the advent of prostaglandins (PG) missed abortion or intrauterine fetal death (IUFD) presented a management dilemma (Lauersen *et al.*, 1980). The conservative approach was to await the start of spontaneous labor, which occurred in 75 % of the patients within 2–3 weeks following the death of the fetus (Tricomi and Kohl, 1957). Failure of spontaneous labor is associated with:

(1) a time-related risk of development of consumptive coagulopathy;
(2) intrauterine infection and septicemia due to introduction of pathogens into the uterine cavity; and
(3) mental distress which may accompany fetal death.

Attempts to induce expulsion of the fetus by oestrogen therapy or oxytocin in high concentrations have generally shown poor results (Embrey *et al.*, 1974).

Since demonstration of the labor-inducing properties of PG in the human myometrium (Karim *et al.*, 1968) PGs have been used successfully to terminate pregnancies complicated by fetal death (Karim *et al.*, 1979).

In an effort to find an optimum dosage regimen, and to reduce side effects, several methods of application of PG have been tried (review by Karim *et al.*, 1979).

Systematic administration of PGs leads from primary labor to cervix dilatation and finally to expulsion of the fetus (Karim, 1970). Cervical rigidity is often an important limiting factor for successful therapy (Brabec *et al.*, 1979). The extra-amniotic application of PGs has shown promising results both for ripening of the cervix and for induction of labor (review by MacKenzie, 1981). Intracervical instillation of PG in a viscous gel aims at administering PG as near as possible to the target organ in order to soften and dilate the cervix (Ulmsten, 1979).

INTRACERVICAL APPLICATION OF PG GEL

The intracervical application of PG gel has been successfully employed either for ripening the cervix prior to surgical evacuation of the uterus during first trimester abortions (Kühnle *et al.*, 1977) or for treatment of the unfavorable cervix before induction of labor at term (Steiner *et al.*, 1979). Previous double-blind studies have confirmed that the PG, and not the gel-vehicle *per se* or its application, is responsible for ripening the cervix (Wingerup *et al.*, 1979; Ulmsten, 1979). Due to the high viscosity of gel, the preparation does not escape via the cervical canal (Lippert, 1979).

In a previous study we treated 15 cases of IUFD with a single or repeated intracervical injection of PG gel (Rath *et al.*, 1982). The PG gel consisted of 3 ml Tylose 5% containing 3 mg $PGF_{2\alpha}$ or 0.5 mg PGE_2. In some cases intravenous oxytocin was necessary to augment contractions. The mean induction−abortion interval was 7.4 h, ranging from 1.5 to 13 h. There were no spontaneous or operation-induced cervical lesions. Side effects due to the intracervical application could be held within tolerable limits. Comparable results have been achieved by using a single intracervical injection of 1.0 mg PGE_2 in a viscous gel (Ekman *et al.*, 1980). The single-dose technique successfully induced abortion in 16 patients with missed labor and IUFD. The mean induction−abortion interval was 7.5 h; no severe side effects or complications were observed in any of the patients (Ekman *et al.*, 1980).

EXTRA-AMNIOTIC ADMINISTRATION OF PG

The extra-amniotic administration of PG, either by a continuous infusion (Embrey *et al.*, 1974; Calder *et al.*, 1976) or by a single or repeated injection of PG gel (Modly and Lippert, 1975; Lippert and Lüthi, 1978) is proven an efficient and safe method for treatment of IUFD. Embrey *et al.* (1974) gave repeated injections or constant infusions of PGE_2 into the extra-amniotic space in cases of missed abortion and IUFD. Induction times were 8−14 h, the dose of PGE_2 required varied from 0.2 to 3.9 mg. These results were confirmed by Calder *et al.* (1976) using the extra-amniotic method in 50 patients with IUFD. The mean induction−abortion interval was 12.5 h.

Repeated extra-amniotic injections of PGE_2 gel have shown comparable results. The main advantage of administered PG in a medium of high viscosity is the greatly delayed PG release (MacKenzie *et al.*, 1977; Lippert, 1979). In the study of Lippert and Lüthi (1978) 20 patients with IUFD were treated with extra-amniotically applied PGE_2 gel. The average induction−abortion interval was 12 h; a mean total dose of 3.8 mg PGE_2 was necessary to terminate pregnancies.

Heinzl (1978) administered 0.5 mg PGE_2 or 5 mg $PGF_{2\alpha}$ in a viscous gel at 2−4 h intervals into the extra-amniotic space in 39 cases of missed abortion and IUFD. The success rates were 92−100% and the mean induction−abortion intervals ranged from 8.0 to 12.5 h. Cervical rupture occurred in one patient with a rigid cervix.

Other studies have confirmed the high efficacy of extra-amniotically applied

PG. The success rates were 100 % and the mean induction–abortion intervals ranged from 8.6 to 10.2 h (Scher *et al.*, 1980; Tsalacopoulos, 1978). Apart from the high efficacy the extra-amniotic method presents additional advantages:

(1) low doses of PGs are required to produce effect (Lippert, 1979); and
(2) gastrointestinal side effects are markedly less frequent and less troublesome than with systemic PG administration (Lippert and Lüthi, 1978).

The disadvantage of extra-amniotic PG application is that it is an invasive technique with a potentially greater risk of intrauterine infection (MacKenzie, 1981); in fact pelvic or intrauterine infection has rarely shown to be a complication of PG administered by this route (Embrey *et al.*, 1974; Lippert and Lüthi, 1978).

COMBINED INTRACERVICAL AND EXTRA-AMNIOTIC PG APPLICATION

The cervix softening and dilating effect of intracervically administered PGF$_{2\alpha}$/PGE$_2$ gel was combined with the labor-inducing property of extra-amniotic PG in 52 patients with IUFD (Rath *et al.*, 1982). Eight to ten hours after intracervical application of PG gel labor was induced either by a continuous extra-amniotic infusion of PGE$_2$ (dose: 100–200 μg/h) or by a single injection of 3–6 mg PGF$_{2\alpha}$ gel or 0.5–1.0 mg PGE$_2$ gel into the extra-amniotic space. Prior to induction of labor epidural anesthesia was performed in all patients. The average total time of therapy, i.e. the interval from intracervical injection of PG gel to expulsion of the fetus, was 27.9 h (range: 16.0–36.0 h) in patients treated with a continuous extra-amniotic infusion, and 18.7 h (range: 4.0–32.0 h) in the extra-amniotic gel-treated group.

The induction of labor to abortion intervals ranged from 2.0 to 12.0 h with a mean of 8.8 h in patients treated with an extra-amniotic PG infusion. The average total dose of extra-amniotically applied PG was 0.97 mg PGE$_2$. In the extra-amniotic PG gel-treated group the mean induction of labor to abortion interval was 7.4 h, ranging from 2.0 to 14.0 h. On an average a total dose of 5 mg PGF$_{2\alpha}$ or 1.0 mg PGE$_2$ was necessary to induce abortion.

No cervical lesions or uterine lacerations were observed in any of the patients. Nausea and vomiting occurred in a total of five cases; blood loss of more than 500 ml due to incomplete expulsion of the placenta was measured in four patients; however, blood transfusions were not necessary. In two cases there were clinical indications of endometritis, otherwise hospitalization was free of fever or complications.

Epidural anesthesia proved to be a gentle and easily regulated method for analgesia in all patients. In comparison with the extra-amniotic PG application the combined intracervical and extra-amniotic PG treatment requires a lower dose of PG for induction of labor. Pretreatment of the cervix reduces the number of extra-amniotic injections necessary, and thus minimizes the risk of intrauterine infection.

Cervical rupture due to labor with a rigid cervix can be avoided by ripening the cervix prior to induction of labor. The success rate of combined PG treatment was 100 %; all patients were delivered vaginally within 24 h after induction of labor.

OTHER ROUTES OF PG APPLICATION

Intravenous route

Administration of prostaglandins by continuous intravenous infusion compares favorably with alternative forms of treatment with respect to efficacy and safety (Karim, 1970; Filshie, 1971).

In general, however, the limiting factors of the intravenous route are the risk of development of painful erythema at the injection site, the relative severity of gastrointestinal side effects and the possibility of uterine hypertonus (Stephens and Birnholz, 1976).

Although later, in cases of IUFD, labor was still induced by means of intravenous administration (Moe, 1976) sometimes in combination with oxytocin (Naismith and Barr, 1974) other forms of application have been employed aiming to reduce the occurrence of undesirable side effects.

Vaginal route

The use of PG vaginal suppositories (20 mg PGE_2) for management of IUFD is highly successful and presents advantages, especially the ease of administration and the absence of uterine invasion (Thiery et al., 1979). Additionally the vaginal route of administration allows removal of drug residues if there are side effects and the patient can remain ambulant during treatment (Southern et al., 1978).

Bailey et al. (1975) presented the first series utilizing PGE_2 suppositories for management of IUFD. They achieved a 100 % success rate, the treatment—delivery interval was a mean of 8.7 h. Results of multicenter clinical trials with this method showed an overall efficacy of 97 % (Southern and Gutknecht, 1976; Southern et al., 1978).

In other studies reported the success rates varied from 92 % to 100 %; the mean induction—abortion intervals ranged from 7.9 to 11.3 h (Kent and Goldstein, 1976; Schulman et al., 1979).

The vaginal instillation of PGE_2 in viscous gel has also been shown to be effective in the management of IUFD (MacKenzie et al., 1979).

Due to poor absorption from the vagina this route requires 25 times more PGE_2 for successful therapy than the extra-amniotic application of PGE_2 (Scher et al., 1980). In comparison with the extra-amniotic route gastrointestinal side effects occurred three to four times more frequently (Scher et al., 1980); pyrexia was observed in 15–63 % of the cases (Schulman et al., 1979; El Demarawy et al., 1977), whereas pyrexia did not occur with the extra-amniotic administration of PG (Scher et al., 1980).

This has been considered such a major drawback that PGE$_2$ suppositories have not been made available on a commercial basis (Thiery et al., 1979).

An additional disadvantage with the vaginal method is that absorption is unpredictable, especially after the membranes rupture or if there is vaginal bleeding (Kent and Goldstein, 1976).

As described with the intra-amniotic (Wentz et al., 1973) and the intravenous administration of PGF$_{2\alpha}$ (Moe, 1976) uterine or cervical rupture in conjunction with the use of PGE$_2$ vaginal suppositories has been reported (Sandler et al., 1979).

Intramuscular route

Clinical evaluation showed that 15-methyl analogs of PGE$_2$ and PGF$_{2\alpha}$ were more potent and had a prolonged uterine stimulatory effect in comparison with natural PGE$_2$ and PGF$_{2\alpha}$ (Toppozada et al., 1972).

Repeated intramuscular injections of 125–500 μg of a 15-methyl PGF$_{2\alpha}$ analog were successful in terminating pregnancies complicated by IUFD in 86–100% of the cases (Boes, 1980; Lange and Secher, 1977). The mean induction–abortion intervals ranged from 7 to 11 h (Ylikorkala et al., 1976; Wallenburg et al., 1980). The advantages with the intramuscular method are the ease of administration and the possibility of individualizing dosage in contrast to the intrauterine methods (Lange and Secher, 1977). On the other hand, the desired aim of inducing labor with a single injection has not been realized. Despite prophylactic or therapeutic medication gastrointestinal side effects were experienced in approximately 90% of the patients (Wallenburg et al., 1980); cases of low uterine rupture in conjunction with this method have been reported (Lange and Secher, 1977).

THE USE OF SULPROSTONE IN CASES OF IUFD

The systemic (intravenous, intramuscular) administration of Sulprostone, a tissue-selective PGE$_2$ derivative, is a promising alternative to other modes of PG application. The success rate depends largely on the route of administration. Extra-amniotic or intracervical application of Sulprostone has shown to be less effective than systemic administration (Schmidt-Gollwitzer et al., 1979; Lippert and Briel, 1980). Several studies have confirmed the high efficacy of Sulprostone administered intravenously or intramuscularly in treatment of IUFD (Gruber and Baumgarten, 1980; Saarikoski et al., 1980). According to these reports abortion was achieved in 86–100% of the cases. The mean induction–abortion intervals ranged from 7 to 13 h. The main advantages of Sulprostone over natural prostaglandins and PG derivatives are lower rates of gastrointestinal side effects and the longer half-life because of slower metabolism (Hess et al., 1977). However, cervical rigidity was reported to be a limiting factor even during systemic administration of Sulprostone; in such cases hysterotomy had been necessary to terminate pregnancy (Brabec et al., 1979).

CONCLUDING REMARKS

All modes of administration of PG have disadvantages; some are complicated and time-consuming, others are associated with a relatively high rate of side effects. The combined intracervical and extra-amniotic application of PG gel is proven an efficient and safe method for treatment of IUFD. It presents several advantages: low dose of PG required, low rates of undesirable side effects and relatively short induction–abortion times. In some cases a single intracervical application of PG gel is sufficient to induce abortion. Infection is rarely a complication of PG administration by this route, and there is no need to resort to antibiotic therapy. Pretreatment of the cervix by intracervically applied PG gel reduces the number of extra-amniotic injections necessary, and thus minimizes the risk of intrauterine infection.

The period of potentially painful contractions can be markedly reduced. Intracervical PGs induce cervical maturation which is similar to the physiological maturation around the time of delivery (Theobald *et al.*, 1982). Thus, ripening of the cervix prior to induction of labor may decrease the failure rate due to a rigid cervix, and minimize the necessity for surgical intervention to terminate pregnancy. It may help to avoid cervical ruptures or lesions and to decrease the likelihood of cervical incompetence in subsequent pregnancies.

References

Bailey, C. D., Newman, C., Ellinas, S. P. and Anderson, G. G. (1975). Use of prostaglandin E_2 vaginal suppositories in intrauterine fetal death and missed abortion. *Obstet. Gynecol.*, **45**, 110–13

Boes, E. G. M. (1980). Missed abortion, hydatidiform mole and intrauterine fetal death treated with 15-methyl-prostaglandin. *S. Afr. Med. J.*, **58**, 878–80

Brabec, W., Dapunt, O. and Bichler, A. (1979). Clinical experiences with Sulprostone. In Schering, A. G. (ed.) *Internationales Sulprostone-Symposium*. Wien. pp. 135–9.

Calder, A. A., MacKenzie, I. Z. and Embrey, M. P. (1976). Intrauterine (extraamniotic) prostaglandins in the management of unsuccessful pregnancy. *J. Reprod. Med.*, **16**, 271–5

Ekman, G., Forman, A., Ulmsten, U. and Wingerup, L. (1980). Termination of pregnancy in patients with missed abortion and intrauterine dead fetuses by a single intracervical application of prostaglandin E_2 in viscous gel. *Zbl. Gynäkol.*, **102**, 219–22

El-Demarawy, H., El-Sahwi, S. and Toppozada, M. K. (1977). Management of missed abortion and fetal death in utero. *Prostaglandins*, **14**, 583–90

Embrey, M. P., Calder, A. A. and Hillier, K. (1974). Extraamniotic prostaglandin in the management of intrauterine fetal death, anencephaly and hydatidiform mole. *J. Obstet. Gynaecol. Br. Commonw.*, **81**, 47–51

Filshie, G. M. (1971). The use of prostaglandin E_2 in the management of intrauterine death, missed abortion and hydatidiform mole. *J. Obstet. Gynaecol. Br. Commonw.*, **78**, 87–90

Gruber, W. S. and Baumgarten, K. (1980). Intravenous prostaglandin E_2 and 16-phenoxy prostaglandin E_2 methyl sulfonamide for induction of fetal death in utero. *Am. J. Obstet. Gynecol.*, **137**, 8–14

Heinzl, S. (1978). Therapeutic abortions in the second trimester of pregnancy with prostaglandin gel. *Geburtsh. Frauenheilk.*, **38**, 220–6

Hess, H. J., Bindra, J. S., Constantine, J. W., Elger, W., Loge, O., Schillinger, E. and Losert, W. (1977). Pharmacology of 16-phenoxy-w-tetranor PGE_2-methyl sulfonamide, a tissue-selective antifertility prostaglandin. *IRCS Med. Sci.*, **5**, 68–75

Karim, S. M. M. (1970). The use of prostaglandin E$_2$ in the management of missed abortion, missed labour and hydatidiform mole. *Br. Med. J.*, **3**, 196–7

Karim, S. M. M., Ng., S. C. and Ratnam, S. S. (1979). Termination of abnormal intrauterine pregnancy with prostaglandins. In Karim, S. M. M. (ed.) *Advances in Prostaglandins Research, Practical Application of Prostaglandins and their Synthesis Inhibitors.* pp. 319–74. (Lancaster: MTP Press)

Karim, S. M. M., Trussel, R. R., Patel, R. C. and Hillier, K. (1968). Response of pregnant human uterus to prostaglandin F$_{2\alpha}$ induction of labor. *Br. Med. J.*, **4**, 621–3

Kent, D. R. and Goldstein, A. J. (1976). Prostaglandin E$_2$ induction of labour for fetal demise. *Obstet. Gynecol.*, **48**, 475–8

Kühnle, H., Grande, P. and Kuhn, W. (1977). Vermeidung dilatationsbedingter Komplikationen beim Schwangerschaftsabbruch durch intrazervikale Applikation eines prostaglandinhaltigen Gels. *Geburtsh. Frauenheilk.*, **37**, 675–80

Lange, A. P. and Secher, W. J. (1977). Midtrimester and missed abortion treated with intramuscular 15(S)-15-methyl-PGF$_2\alpha$. *Prostaglandins*, **14**, 389–95

Lauersen, N. H., Cederqvist, L. L. and Wilson, K. H. (1980). Management of intrauterine fetal death with prostaglandin E$_2$ vaginal suppositories. *Obstet. Gynecol.*, **137**, 753–7

Lippert, T. H. (1979). The use of prostaglandin gel in obstetrics and gynecology. *Arch. Gynecol.*, **227**, 171–9

Lippert, T. H. and Briel, R. C. (1980). The use of sulprostone, a prostaglandin E$_2$ derivate, in intrauterine fetal death and therapeutic abortion. *Prostaglandins Med.*, **5**, 259–65

Lippert, T. H. and Lüthi, A. (1978). Induction of labour with prostaglandin E$_2$ gel in cases of intrauterine fetal death. *Prostaglandins*, **15**, 533–42

MacKenzie, I. Z. (1981). Clinical studies on cervical ripening. In Ellwood, D. A. and Anderson, A. B. M. (eds.) *The Human Cervix in Pregnancy and Labour.* pp. 163–86. (Edinburgh, London, Melbourne, New York: Churchill Livingstone)

MacKenzie, I. Z., Davies, A. J. and Embrey, M. P. (1979). Fetal death in utero managed with vaginal prostaglandin E$_2$ gel. *Br. Med. J.*, **1**, 1764–5

MacKenzie, I. Z., Dilley, S. and Embrey, M. P. (1977). The kinetics of extra-amniotically injected prostaglandins to induce midtrimester abortion. *Prostaglandins*, **13**, 975–86

Modly, T. and Lippert, T. H. (1975). Prostaglandin-Gel zur Abortinduktion und Geburtseinleitung bei intrauterinem Fruchttod. *Arch. Gynecol.*, **219**, 498–9

Moe, N. (1976). The intravenous infusion of prostaglandin F$_{2\alpha}$ in the management of intrauterine death of the fetus. *Acta Obstet. Gynecol Scand.*, **55**, 113–14

Naismith, W. C. M. K. and Barr, W. (1974). Simultaneous intravenous infusion of prostaglandin E$_2$ (PGE$_2$) and oxytocin in the management of intrauterine death of the fetus, missed abortion and hydatidiform mole. *J. Obstet. Gynaecol. Br. Commonw.*, **81**, 146–9

Rath, W., Kühnle, H., Theobald, P. and Kuhn, W. (1982). Geburtseinleitung beim intrauterinen Fruchttod mittels intrazervikaler und extraamnialer Prostaglandinapplikation. *Gynäkol. Prax.*, **6**, 713–17

Saarikoski, S., Selander, K. and Pystynen, P. (1980). Induction of labour with sulprostone after foetal death and in hydatidiform mole. *Prostaglandins*, **20**, 481–5

Sandler, R. Z., Knutzen, V. K., Milano, Ch. M. and Gleichner, W. (1979). Uterine rupture with the use of vaginal prostaglandin E$_2$ suppositories. *Am. J. Obstet. Gynecol.*, **134**, 348–9

Scher, J., Dai-Yun Jeng, Moshirpur, J. and Kerenyi, T. D. (1980). A comparison between vaginal prostaglandin E$_2$ suppositories and intrauterine extra-amniotic prostaglandins in the management of fetal death in utero. *Am. J. Obstet. Gynecol.*, **137**, 769–72

Schmidt-Gollwitzer, K., Schüssler, B., Elger, W. and Schmidt-Gollwitzer, M. (1979). A new therapeutic approach for terminating intact and disturbed pregnancies. Three years of experience with the prostaglandin E$_2$ derivate sulprostone. *Geburtsh. Frauenheilk.*, **39**, 667–75

Schulman, H., Saldana, L., Chin-Chu, L. and Randolph, G. (1979). Mechanism of failed labor after fetal death and its treatment with prostaglandin E$_2$. *Am. J. Obstet. Gynecol.*, **133**, 742–52

Southern, E. M. and Gutknecht, G. D. (1976). Management of intrauterine fetal demise and missed abortion using prostaglandin E$_2$ vaginal suppositories. *Obstet. Gynecol.*, **47**, 602–6

Southern, E. M., Gutknecht, G. D., Mohberg, N. R. and Edelman, D. A. (1978). Vaginal prostaglandin E$_2$ in the management of fetal intrauterine death. *Br. J. Obstet. Gynaecol.*, **85**, 437–41

Steiner, H., Zahradnik, H. P., Breckwoldt, M., Robrecht, D. and Hillemanns, H. G. (1979).

Cervical ripening prior to induction of labour (intra-cervical application of PGE_2 viscous gel). *Prostaglandins*, **17**, 125–33

Stephens, J. D. and Birnholz, J. C. (1976). Modern management of fetal death in utero and missed abortion. In Karim, S. M. M. (ed.) *Obstetric and Gynaecological Uses of Prostaglandins*. pp. 253–9. (Lancaster: MTP Press)

Theobald, P., Rath, W., Kühnle, H. and Kuhn, W. (1982). Histological and electron-microscopic examinations of collagenous tissue of the non-pregnant cervix, the pregnant cervix and the pregnant prostaglandin-treated cervix. *Arch. Gynecol.*, **231**, 241–5

Thiery, M., Amy, J. J. and Decoster, J. M. (1979). Vaginal prostaglandin E_2 for interruption of pregnancy and management of intrauterine death. *Z. Geburtsh. Perinat.*, **183**, 218–22

Toppozada, M. K., Beguin, J., Bydgeman, M. and Wiqvist, N. (1972). Response of the midpregnant human uterus to systemic administration of 15(S)-15-methyl-prostaglandin $F_{2\alpha}$. *Prostaglandins*, **2**, 239–44

Tricomi, V. and Kohl, S. G. (1975). Fetal death in utero. *Am. J. Obstet. Gynecol.*, **74**, 1092–7

Tsalacopoulos, G. (1978). Intrauterine extra-amniotic prostaglandin $F_{2\alpha}$ in the management of patients with intra-uterine fetal death. *S. Afr. Med. J.*, **53**, 848–52

Ulmsten, U. (1979). Aspects on ripening of the cervix and induction of labor by intracervical application of PGE_2 in viscous gel. *Acta Obstet. Gynecol. Scand.*, Suppl. 84, 5–9

Wallenburg, H. C. S., Keirse, M. J. N. C., Freie, H. M. P. and Blaquiere, J. F. (1980). Intramuscular administration of 15(S)-15-methyl-prostaglandin $F_{2\alpha}$ for induction of labour in patients with fetal death. *Br. J. Obstet. Gynaecol.*, **87**, 203–9

Wentz, A. C., Thompson, B. E. and King, T. M. (1973). Posterior cervical rupture following prostaglandin-induced mid-trimester abortion. *Am. J. Obstet. Gynecol.*, **115**, 1107–10

Wingerup, L., Ulmsten, U. and Andersson, K.-E. (1979). Ripening of the cervix by intracervical application of PGE_2-gel before termination of pregnancy with dilatation and evacuation. *Acta Obstet. Gynecol. Scand.*, Suppl. 84, 15–18

Ylikorkala, O., Kirkinen, P. and Järvinen, P. A. (1976). Intramuscular adminsitration of 15-methyl-prostaglandin $F_{2\alpha}$ for induction of labour in patients with intrauterine fetal death or an anencephalic fetus. *Br. J. Obstet. Gynaecol.*, **83**, 502–4

6

Extra-amniotic prostaglandins for second trimester abortion

M. P. EMBREY and I. Z. MACKENZIE

The extra-amniotic technique of prostaglandin administration for induction of abortion was first introduced in the early 1970s (Wiqvist and Bygdeman, 1970; Embrey and Hillier, 1971) since when the method has gained increasing popularity as a reliable method for termination of second trimester pregnancies especially during the range 13–16 weeks gestation when intra-amniotic methods are frequently technically difficult. During the course of the past 12 years many different protocols have been investigated, the aim being the development of a single-injection procedure using the lowest effective dose of prostaglandin to achieve abortion within a reasonable time interval (less than 36 h) with minimal side effects and risks to the patient. In pursuit of these goals, various injection techniques have been explored using both the natural prostaglandins alone or in combination with other oxytocics or aborti-facients, or using one of the newer prostaglandin analogs. As well as studies conducted to improve administration methods and efficacy, analyses have been made of associated morbidity and long-term sequelae that might result from abortion induced this way.

ADMINISTRATION PROTOCOLS

The initial reports by Wiqvist and Bygdeman (1970) and Embrey and Hillier (1971) indicated that the extra-amniotic administration of repeated small doses of PGE_2 or $PGF_{2\alpha}$ is an effective means of provoking abortion comparing favorably with intravenous administration. Larger studies confirmed the original observations that 2-hourly injections of PGE_2 200 μg or $PGF_{2\alpha}$ 750 μg were appropriate doses, while the use of a self-retaining Foley catheter to facilitate the repeated instillations was recommended (Embrey and Hillier, 1971). By adding a concomitant intravenous infusion of oxytocin to the extra-amniotic regimen (Embrey et al., 1973), and utilizing the enhancement effect noted between prostaglandins and oxytocin (Brummer, 1971; Gillespie, 1972) the efficacy of the technique could be improved. Mean injection–abortion intervals were consequently shortened to approximately 15 h. As an alternative to intermittent hourly or 2-hourly injections, continuous infusions using an automatic infusion pump were tried, producing essentially similar results (Miller et al., 1972; Midwinter et al., 1972).

In 1973 Lippert and Modly introduced the concept of combining prostaglandins into a viscous gel to be injected at 3-hourly intervals and this vehicle was further explored by MacKenzie et al. (1975a), who developed the principle of a single extra-amniotic injection technique using the natural prostaglandins. These workers showed that this single injection of PGE_2 1.5 mg in a 5 % aqueous solution of methyl-hydroxyethyl cellulose (Tylose) would successfully induce abortion within 24 h in 75 % of cases: larger does of PGE_2 did not increase efficiency while $PGE_{2\alpha}$ 10 mg was less effective (MacKenzie and Embrey, 1976). The presence of a self-retaining catheter did not appear to influence these results. Other variants of the extra-amniotic technique have also been proposed. These include combinations with extra-amniotic solutions, normal saline, hypertonic saline and rivanol (Ölund and Larsson, 1978). These latter combinations have all had the main aim of developing a single-injection procedure while maintaining previously achieved efficacy. In general, however, results have been marginally less impressive, probably due to the tendency for the abortifacient solution to leak through the cervical os, possibly due to the large volumes of fluid required. To augment prostaglandin activity and shorten abortion times other alternative approaches have been used, including the insertion of laminaria tents (Hodgson, 1979) and intra-amniotic administration of hyperosmolar saline or urea solutions (Craft, 1982). There is some risk of adverse effects, e.g. hypernatremia, and coagulopathy with hypertonic solutions which may be reserved to ensure non-viability of the fetus in later abortions.

Gastrointestinal side effects are likely to occur with all methods of extra-amniotic administration and appear to be dose-related. With PGE_2 vomiting occurs in 25–40 % of cases and diarrhea in 5–20 %, while with $PGF_{2\alpha}$ incidences are slightly higher at 40–55 % and 15–30 % respectively. Other side effects are uncommon with both prostaglandins due to the relatively low doses required to induce abortion compared with all other administration routes.

Research over the past decade has resulted in the synthesis of analogs exhibiting enhanced utero-tonic specificity and greater resistance to metabolic degradation. Formulated to inactivate C15 dehydrogenation are the 15-methyl and 16,16-dimethyl derivatives of PGE_2 and $PGF_{2\alpha}$ and some related compounds. Both types of compounds have been studied clinically, and both have their limitations. The frequency of side effects caused by 15-methyl analogs limits their usefulness, especially if given systemically. The 16,16-dimethyl compounds have greater uterine specificity but their lack of chemical stability is a drawback.

MECHANISM OF ACTION

The precise mechanism of action by which extra-amniotically injected prostaglandins affect abortion remains speculative. Gustavii and Green (1972) studied the effect of extra-amniotic injections of hypertonic saline given to induce abortion and observed increased production of prostaglandins by both decidua and fetal membranes which they postulated reached the myometrium stimulating contractions and thus abortion. Exogenous prostaglandin injections presumably produce the same result, both by direct action upon the myometrium and by provoking the release of endogenous prostaglandins. The continued presence of the prostaglandins, once injected into the extra-amniotic space, appears to be important. Radiographic studies, using radio-opaque dyes, combined with saline and prostaglandin solutions have illustrated the rapidity of the removal of the injected solution from the chorio-decidual space (Wiqvist et al., 1972; Dillon et al., 1974; MacKenzie et al., 1977) and led to the suggestion that fundal placement of the catheter might improve results (Braaksma et al., 1972; Csapo et al., 1972; Read et al., 1974). It was, however, the authors' experience – and that of Wiqvist et al. (1972) – that unnecessary advancement of the catheter to the uterine fundus was more likely to cause bleeding into the catheter lumen due to trauma of the decidua with consequent sudden absorption of prostaglandins into the systemic circulation, leading to an acute reaction experienced by the patient in the form of pallor, hypotension and severe pelvic pain. These latter observations supported the view that the combination of prostaglandins with a viscous medium would reduce the rate of absorption of prostaglandins from the extra-amniotic space, thereby reducing the incidence of acute reaction and hopefully allowing the prostaglandins to remain in the extra-amniotic space for a prolonged period, permitting a single-injection technique. Further studies analyzing the release of injected prostaglandins in viscous gel into the amniotic fluid and peripheral blood indicated that this release vehicle did produce a slower uptake (MacKenzie et al., 1977).

REPORTED RESULTS

Table 6.1 lists results from selected published series using different protocols of extra-amniotic injection of the natural prostaglandins and those using some

Table 6.1 Selected series of results of induction of abortion using the natural prostaglandins and prostaglandin analogs

| Reference | PG used, and protocol | Cases treated | Percentage abortion in | | Mean induction– abortion interval (h) |
			24 h	36 h	
Embrey et al., 1973	$F_{2\alpha}$ 750 µg: 2 hourly	93		79	24.9
Fylling and Refsdal, 1974	$F_{2\alpha}$: 5 mg	100	81		12.4
Fraser and Brash, 1974	E_2 100–200 µg: hourly	104		89	18.3
MacKenzie and Embrey, 1976	E_2: 1.5–2.0 mg	166	75		16.4
Karim, 1976	$2_\alpha, 2_\beta$-dihomo-15meF$_{2\alpha}$: 1 mg	316	82		14.5
WHO, 1977	15 me-F$_{2\alpha}$: 0.92 mg	660		80	16.2
Tejuja et al., 1978	15 me-F$_{2\alpha}$: 1 mg	1569		78	14.8
Kunz et al., 1979	16-Phenoxy-PGE$_2$-methyl-sulfonamide: 100 mg	121	82		11.0
Embrey and MacKenzie, 1980, unpublished communication	16, 16-diMe-E$_2$: 1.0 mg	29	72		18:2

of the analogs which have been studied using the extra-amniotic injection technique.

The general conclusion may be made that despite the development of longer-acting selective utero-tonic prostaglandins, results with these compounds in terms of efficacy and side effects are not significantly better than those achieved with the natural prostaglandin PGE_2 in combination with a continuous intravenous infusion of oxytocin.

ASSOCIATED MORBIDITY

As with other methods of inducing late abortion, the extra-amniotic injection of prostaglandins may result in complications. Compared with the numbers of reports assessing the efficiency of different administration protocols and dosages, relatively little attention has been paid to associated morbidity.

Hemorrhage in excess of 500 ml occurring at the time of abortion is generally more frequent with mid-trimester than first-trimester abortions. Between 12 and 22 weeks gestation, however, a direct relationship does not exist; approximately $1-2\%$ of all such cases are complicated by excessive hemorrhage (MacKenzie, 1981). Few studies have compared the incidence of hemorrhage following extra-amniotic therapy with the intra-amniotic route, and analyses of results obtained in different units can lead to spurious, unreliable conclusions. Fraser and Brash (1974) noted no difference between administration routes, and MacKenzie (1981) reached a similar conclusion.

Incomplete abortion requiring completion by surgical evacuation is a function of gestation rather than the protocol of prostaglandin administration. Figure 6.1 illustrates the relationship with gestation, indicating that 50% of abortions induced between 11 and 12 weeks gestation are incomplete, reducing to 10% of those performed at 19 weeks gestation and over. However,

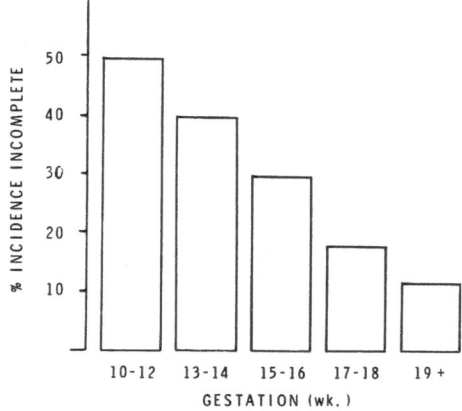

Fig. 6.1 The incidence of incomplete abortion following extra-amniotic injection of prostaglandin to induce abortion related to the gestational period at the time of abortion

when the abortion is incomplete, general anesthesia, with its attendant potential morbidity, is frequently necessary and excessive bleeding and post-abortal sepsis is more common. The frequency with which post-abortion intrauterine sepsis occurs is, however, obscure. Personal experience (MacKenzie and Fry, 1981; MacKenzie, 1981) has shown that 1 % of patients undergoing a late first or second trimester abortion induced by extra-amniotic prostaglandins were given antibiotics because of a pyrexia during the procedure or in the post-abortal period, or as a prophylactic maneuver while only 0.05–0.3 % developed overt sepsis. Reassessment 6 weeks post-abortion indicated that 2.6 % had complained of symptoms consistent with sepsis but the diagnosis was only confirmed in 0.2 %. Patients at particular risk appeared to be those with prolonged abortion times (more than 24 h), and incomplete expulsion of the placenta. The results are similar to those obtained with intra-amniotic prostaglandin therapy (MacKenzie, 1981).

Genital tract trauma following mid-trimester extra-amniotic prostaglandin treatment alone is uncommon. Sporadic reports of uterine rupture have appeared in the literature (Smith, 1975; Duenhoelter and Gant, 1975; Emery et al., 1979) but the number following extra-amniotic therapy is small compared with the reports following intra-amniotic and vaginal therapy: however, since the total numbers treated by the different routes are not known, worthwhile comparisons are not possible. Cervical rupture, or cervico-vaginal fistulae, also seem to occur less frequently following extra-amniotic therapy than with intra-amniotic therapy, but again such conclusions must be tenuous due to uncertain denominators for different administration routes. However, this conclusion seems reasonable if one postulates that the prostaglandins are placed in the lower uterine pole with extra-amniotic therapy, and can have a direct cervical softening effect, thus reducing the chances of a firm, rigid cervix resisting effacement and dilatation. Further, if a self-retaining Foley catheter is used as part of the treatment method the balloon and catheter may protect against fetal expulsion through the posterior vaginal fornix.

Other specific complications occurring as an immediate or early consequence of an extra-amniotic prostaglandin-induced abortion, notably a consumptive coagulopathy or epileptiform seizures, have now been largely eliminated. Studies on coagulation changes have indicated that the prostaglandins alone, however administered, do not alter coagulation homeostasis (Badraoui et al., 1973; MacKenzie et al., 1975b) but if given in combination with a hypertonic solution, a coagulopathy may develop (Burnett et al., 1975; MacKenzie et al., 1975; Grundy and Craven, 1976).

Thromboembolism was a major cause of maternal death in the United Kingdom during the first few years following the passing of the 1967 Abortion Act. Several factors have contributed to the reduced incidence of this complication. In the Oxford series, for example, by refining the method of extra-amniotic prostaglandin administration using a viscous gel and combining the additive effect of concomitant intravenous infusion of oxytocin, so shortening the induction/abortion intervals, the length of hospital stay has been considerably reduced (Table 6.2). Reduction in the need for general anesthesia, using a selective policy for surgical evacuation based on examination of the products passed and a pelvic examination indicating incomplete

Table 6.2 The duration of hospital admission using three different protocols of extra-amniotic (EA) PGE$_2$ injection developed in Oxford during the past 10 years: in all instances a concomitant intravenous infusion of oxytocin is given

	Intermittent 200 μg PGE$_2$ EA injection (%)	Single 1.5 mg PGE$_2$ EA injection (%)	Single 2.5 mg PGE$_2$ EA injection (%)
1 night	26	55	71
2 nights	49	38	26
3 or more nights	25	7	3

abortion, has also helped to reduce hospital stay and thus lessen the risk of thromboembolism. Of 1730 patients treated in Oxford with extra-amniotic prostaglandins to induce mid-trimester abortion, the incidence of venous thrombosis has been 0.1 % with no pulmonary emboli occurring.

As with morbidity, relatively little attention has been paid to the early recovery patterns in patients. The duration of uterine bleeding following abortion in 535 women treated with extra-amniotic PGE$_2$, PGF$_{2\alpha}$, or 15-methyl-PGF$_{2\alpha}$, in Oxford (MacKenzie, 1981) is illustrated in Table 6.3. There was no apparent relationship between the gestation at which abortion was performed, or the need for surgical evacuation of an incomplete abortion and the duration of bleeding. Altogether, 2.5 % of patients required re-admission for surgical re-evacuation for vaginal bleeding problems. In the same 535 cases the menstrual cycle was re-established within 4 weeks of abortion in 22 %, between 4 and 6 weeks in 51 % and in more than 6 weeks in 27 %. Again, gestation at abortion, and management of the abortion, did not appear to influence this recovery pattern.

Table 6.3 The duration of uterine bleeding in 535 patients following therapeutic abortion induced with extra-amniotic prostaglandin

Uterine bleeding ceased	< 7 days	12.8 %
	> 21 days	17.6 %
Menstruation returned	< 4 weeks	21.0 %
	> 6 weeks	28.0 %

Breast activity, secretion or lactation is a common occurrence following mid-trimester abortion which does not appear to be related to prostaglandin used or dose given, or the route of prostaglandin administration. Gestation at abortion, however, correlates directly with the incidence of breast activity, as shown in Figure 6.2. In none of the patients reporting this symptom was it a morbid feature.

DELAYED SEQUELAE

Surprisingly, there is still a dearth of information about the long-term effects of a mid-trimester abortion induced with extra-amniotic prostaglandins.

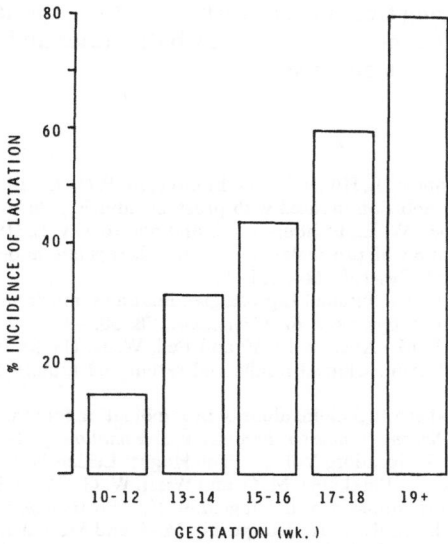

Fig. 6.2 The incidence of lactation following abortion induced with prostaglandins at different gestational periods

Personal studies (MacKenzie and Hillier, 1975; MacKenzie, 1981) assessing morbidity following intra- and extra-amniotic treatment have failed to show any specific ill-health resulting from the previous abortion. Menstrual function and menstrual symptoms have not been found to be provoked by the termination as judged by patient responses given $1\frac{1}{2}$–2 years after the original termination. Similarly, there appears to be no adverse effect on future fertility (MacKenzie and Fry, unpublished data) and the outcome of pregnancies conceived following a mid-trimester prostaglandin-induced abortion (MacKenzie and Hillier, 1977). However, further results are necessary to substantiate these initial observations.

CONCLUSIONS

Clinical experience with the extra-amniotic administration of prostaglandin analogs for pregnancy termination over the past decade has been somewhat disappointing. Of the analogs tested, results generally have not shown great improvement over those initially reported in the early 1970s using the natural prostaglandins. To some extent the comparative lack of progress is due to the fact that greater attention has been directed to simplifying abortion procedures, moving away from the intrauterine methods. However, until significantly improved results are achieved with intravaginal or intramuscular administration techniques, the extra-amniotic route is likely to remain the most popular within the United Kingdom. The dosages required are low, with consequently relatively low side effects, while administration using a viscous gel is simple, allowing treatment as early as 12 weeks gestation with minimal nursing attention required, with low morbidity rates and no specific complications related to the technique.

References

Badraoui, M. H. H., Bonnar, J., Hillier, K. and Embrey, M. P. (1973). Blood coagulation changes during midtrimester abortion induced with prostaglandin $F_{2\alpha}$. *Br. Med. J.*, **4**, 375–8

Braaksma, J. J., Brenner, W. E., Fishburne, J. I. and Staurovsky, L. (1972). Intrauterine extra-amniotic administration of prostaglandin $F_{2\alpha}$ for therapeutic abortion. Early myometrial effects. *Am. J. Obstet. Gynecol.*, **114**, 511–15

Brummer, H. C. (1971). Interaction of E-prostaglandins and syntocinon on the pregnant human myometrium. *J. Obstet. Gynaecol. Br. Commonw.*, **78**, 305–9

Burnett, L. S., King, T. M., Atienza, M. F. and Bell, W. R. (1975). Intra-amniotic urea as a midtrimester abortifacient: Clinical results and serum and urinary changes. *Am. J. Obstet. Gynecol.*, **121**, 7–16

Craft, I. (1982). Natural prostaglandins alone or in combination for termination of pregnancy. In Keirse *et al.* (eds.) *Second Trimester Pregnancy Termination.* p. 108. Boerhaave Series for postgraduate medical education, Vol. 22. (The Hague: Leiden University Press)

Csapo, A. I., Kivikoski, A., Pulkkinen, M. O. and Wiest, W. G. (1972). First trimester abortions induced by extraovular infusion of prostaglandin $F_{2\alpha}$. *Prostaglandins*, **1**, 295–303

Dillon, T. F., Phillips, L. L., Rosk, A., Horiguchit, M.-S. and Mootabar, H. (1974). The efficacy of prostaglandin $F_{2\alpha}$ in second trimester abortion – coagulation and hormonal aspects. *Am. J. Obstet. Gynecol.*, **118**, 688–99

Duenhoelter, J. H. and Gant, N. F. (1975). Complications following prostaglandin $F_{2\alpha}$ induced midtrimester abortion. *Obstet. Gynecol.*, **46**, 247–50

Embrey, M. P. and Hillier, K. (1971). Therapeutic abortion by intrauterine instillation of prostaglandins. *Br. Med. J.*, **1**, 588–90

Embrey, M. P., Hillier, K. and Mahendran, P. (1973). Termination of pregnancy by extra-amniotic prostaglandins and the synergistic action of oxytocin. *Adv. Biosci.*, **9**, 507–13

Emery, S., Jarvis, G. J. and Johnson, D. A. N. (1979). Uterine rupture after intra-amniotic injection of prostaglandin E_2. *Br. Med. J.*, **2**, 51

Fraser, I. S. and Brash, J. H. (1974). Comparison of extra- and intra-amniotic prostaglandins for therapeutic abortion. *Obstet. Gynecol.*, **43**, 97–103

Fylling, P. and Refsdal, A. (1974). Therapeutic abortion by a single extra-amniotic instillation of prostaglandin $F_{2\alpha}$. *Arch. Gynaecol.*, **217**, 119–25

Gillespie, A. (1972). Prostaglandin–oxytocin enhancement and potentiation and their clinical applications. *Br. Med. J.*, **1**, 15–152

Grundy, M. R. and Craven, E. R. (1976). Consumptive coagulopathy after intra-amniotic urea. *Br. Med. J.*, **2**, 677–8

Gustavii, B. and Green, K. (1972). Release of prostaglandin $F_{2\alpha}$ following injection of hypertonic saline for therapeutic abortion: a preliminary study. *Am. J. Obstet. Gynecol.*, **114**, 1099–100

Hodgson, J. E. (1979). Three hundred late midtrimester abortions induced by extra-amniotic PGF_{2A} and intracervical laminaria tests. *Adv. Planned Parenthood*, **14**, 61–7

Karim, S. M. M. (1976). Singapore experience with prostaglandins – routine use and recent advances. In Karim, S. M. M. (ed.) *Obstetric and Gynaecological Uses of Prostaglandins.* pp. 127–54. Proc. of the Asian Federation of Obstetrics and Gynaecological Congress. (Lancaster: MTP Press)

Kunz, J., Kunz-Padrutt, M., Banninger, U., Reich, P. and Keller, P. J. (1979). Abortinduktion im 1. und 2. Trimenon durch extra-amniale instillation eines Prostaglandin E_2-Derivates, *Geburtshilfe Frauenheilkd*, **39**, 798–808

Lippert, T. H. and Modly, T. (1973). Induction of abortion by the extra-amniotic administration of prostaglandin gels. *J. Obstet. Gynaecol. Br. Commonw.*, **80**, 1025–7

MacKenzie, I. Z. (1981). Abortion induced with intrauterine prostaglandins: an assessment of the associated morbidity and early and delayed sequelae. *MD Thesis*, Bristol University

MacKenzie, I. Z. and Embrey, M. P. (1976). Single extra-amniotic injection of prostaglandins in viscous gel to induce abortion. *Br. J. Obstet. Gynaecol.*, **83**, 505–7

MacKenzie, I. Z. and Fry, A. (1981). Postabortal sepsis and antibiotic prophylaxis. *Br. Med. J.,* **282,** 476–7

MacKenzie, I. Z. and Hillier, K. (1975). Delayed morbidity following prostaglandin induced abortion. *Int. J. Obstet. Gynaecol.,* **13,** 209–14

Mackenzie, I. Z. and Hillier, K. (1977). Prostaglandin-induced abortion and outcome of subsequent pregnancies: a prospective controlled study. *Br. Med. J.,* **2,** 1114–17

MacKenzie, I. Z., Dilley, S. and Embrey, M. P. (1977). The kinetics of extra-amniotically injected prostaglandins to induce midtrimester abortion. *Prostaglandins,* **13,** 975–86

MacKenzie, I. Z., Hillier, K. and Embrey, M. P. (1975a). Single extra-amniotic injection of prostaglandin E_2 in viscous gel to induce mid-trimester abortion. *Br. Med. J.,* **1,** 240–2

MacKenzie, I. Z., Sayers, L., Bonnar, J. and Hillier, K. (1975b). Coagulation changes during mid-trimester abortion induced with intra-amniotic prostaglandin E_2 and hypertonic solutions. *Lancet,* **2,** 1066–9

Midwinter, A., Bowen, M. and Shepherd, A. (1972). Continuous intrauterine infusion of prostaglandin E_2 for termination of pregnancy. *J. Obstet. Gynaecol. Br. Commonw.,* **79,** 807–9

Miller, A. W. F., Calder, A. A. and MacNaughton, M. C. (1972). Termination of pregnancy by continuous intrauterine infusion of prostaglandins. *Lancet,* **2,** 5–7

Ölund, A. R. and Larsson, B. (1978). Comparison of extra-amniotic instillation of Rivanol and $PGF_{2\alpha}$, either separately or in combination followed by oxytocin for second trimester abortion. *Acta Obstet. Gynecol. Scand.,* **57,** 333–6

Read, M. D., Bedford, N. A. and Martin, R. H. (1974). Induction of abortion in early second-trimester pregnancy. *Lancet,* **1,** 214

Smith, A. M. (1975). Rupture of uterus during prostaglandin-induced abortion. *Br. Med. J.,* **1,** 205

Tejuja, S., Choudhury, S. D. and Manchanda, P. K. (1978). Use of intra- and extra-amniotic prostaglandins for the termination of pregnancy, Report of Multicentric Trial in India, *Contraception,* **18,** 641–52

World Health Organization Task Force on the use of prostaglandins for the regulation of fertility (1977). Prostaglandins and Abortion: II. single extra-amniotic administration of 0.92 mg of 15-methyl-prostaglandin $F_{2\alpha}$ in Hiskon for termination of pregnancies in weeks 10–20 of gestation: an international multicenter study. *Am. J. Obstet. Gynecol.,* **129,** 597–600

Wiqvist, N. and Bygdeman, M. (1970). Therapeutic abortion by local administration of prostaglandin. *Lancet,* **2,** 716–17

Wiqvist, N., Beguin, F., Bygdeman, M., Fernstrom, I. and Toppozada , M. K. (1972). Induction of abortion by extra-amniotic prostaglandin administration. *Prostaglandins,* **1,** 37–53

7
New prostaglandin delivery systems

M. P. EMBREY

The parturogenic and abortifacient effects of the prostaglandins (PGs) have been extensively investigated over the past decade, and clinical roles and preferable techniques in the induction of labor and abortion defined. Because of their diverse biological effects and rapid degradation systemic absorption of PGs results in significant side effects and consequently methods of local administration have been increasingly adopted.

A particular recent development has been the recognition that PGE_2, by virtue of its cervical softening as well as oxytocic activity, has a valuable role in the induction of labor, especially when the cervix is unripe. Initially administration was intrauterine but vaginal application in simple gels or lipid-based pessaries has been found to be as effective and more convenient. The clinical benefit of the PGE_2 regimen is increasingly recognized and is now used in the majority of units in the UK, but a hindrance to its wider utilization has been the inherent lability of PGE_2, so that the simple gels and pessaries lack adequate long-term stability while they do not provide sustained uniform release.

Partly because similar criticisms apply to the use of PGE analogs in simple pessaries, the prostaglandins have not yet fulfilled their early promise in fertility regulation. Recent studies, while showing the efficacy of PG analogs administered in simple lipid-based (e.g. Witepsol) vaginal pessaries for termination of early pregnancy (menstrual induction) have demonstrated also the limitations of the products currently available – namely that (1) repeated administration is necessary, (2) while PGF analogs mostly cause unacceptable side effects, (3) the clinically superior PGE analogs are unstable and this has deterred development. Clinicians need a packaged product with long-term storage stability providing sustained release of an efficacious PG from a solitary vaginal pessary.

Attempts to overcome these difficulties hitherto have been only partially successful. It was hoped, for example, that the use of a Witepsol pessary with a higher melting point might provide a single-dose delivery vehicle, but experience showed that results were less consistently successful than when administration was repeated (Tejuja *et al.*, 1979). In another approach the PG analog was incorporated in a slow-release Silastic vaginal device. In clinical practice the device was disappointing, one problem being the frequency with which the device was expelled prematurely. Rather than the expected controlled sustained release, absorption from the device was erratic, and trials showed wide variation in success rates and the incidence of side effects (Hendricks *et al.*, 1976; Lauerson and Wilson, 1976).

Recent work has shown that the problem of providing stability and sustained release can be resolved by incorporating the PG in a novel polymer vaginal pessary (suppository) (Embrey *et al.*, 1980).

POLYMER FORMULATIONS

Polyethylene oxide cross-linked polymers, from formulations of moderate molecular weight polyethylene glycol, 1,2,6-hexane triol and pure dicyclohexane methane 4,4′-di-isocyanate, are hydrophilic (hydrogels) and even when swollen to several times their initial dry weight remain tough and rubbery.

The reactants are mixed in stoichiometric proportions at 80 °C and poured into heated Teflon or poly(propylene) moulds to cure at 95 °C. After cooling, the polyethylene oxide hydrogel block is cut to the dimensions required for the pessaries. Residual material of low molecular weight is extracted in water and samples vacuum-dried at room temperature.

The prostaglandin is incorporated in the samples by swelling them in a 1 : 1 w : w chloroform/ethanol solution of the PG, the concentration of the solution being calculated from the required content of the pessary and the equilibrium swelling of the polymer in the solution. The fully swollen pessaries are vacuum-dried to constant weight at ambient temperature, yielding polyethylene oxide pessaries with the PG uniformly dispersed through the matrix.

RELEASE CHARACTERISTICS

The release characteristics of the pessary can be studied *in vitro* by measuring ^3H release in phosphate buffer at 37 °C from a labled pessary (prepared as above) containing prostaglandin and tracer amounts of PGE_2. At regular intervals the buffer solution is replaced and the radioactive content determined by scintillation counting techniques. The release of radioactive PG is expressed as a percentage of the total radioactive content. The dry device, as it swells *in vitro* or *in vivo* with absorption of water and diffusion of PGE_2 across the polymer/fluid interface, shows a reasonably constant release (zero order) over a considerable period before changing to a lower value. Its half-life is directly proportional to the square of the thickness of the device, making it possible to calculate the optimum thickness for a particular half-life giving a desired performance. The *in vitro* release profile of a prostaglandin E_2 polymer pessary is shown in Fig. 7.1. The pessary released approximately 80 % of its content over 12 h and possessed a $t_{\frac{1}{2}}$ of 7.2 h. Its clinical performance in ripening the unfavorable cervix has been previously described (Embrey *et al.*, 1980). The release characteristics of a pessary with a shorter half-life ($t_{\frac{1}{2}} = 3.8$ h) which

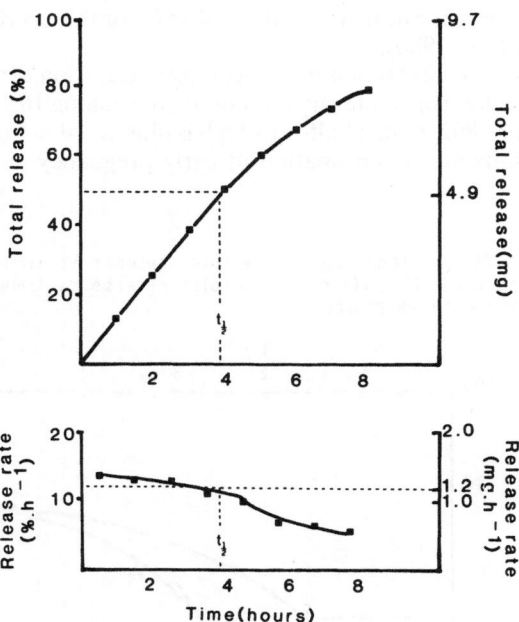

Fig. 7.1 *In vitro* release of prostaglandin E_2 in phosphate buffer at $37\,°C$ ($t_{\frac{1}{2}} = 7.2\,h$).

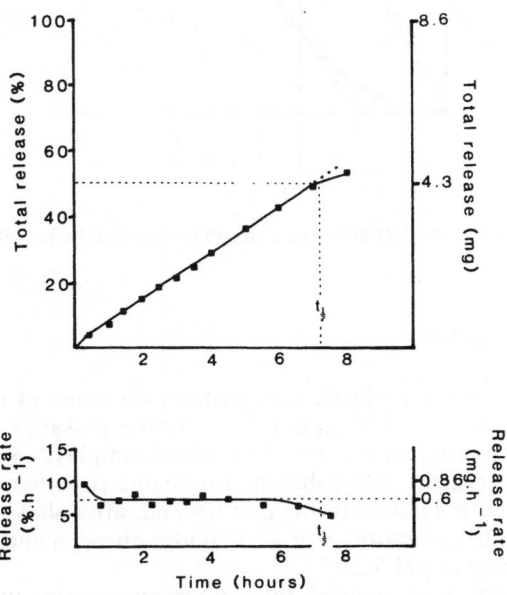

Fig. 7.2 *In vitro* release of prostaglandin E_2 in phosphate buffer at $37\,°C$ ($t_{\frac{1}{2}} = 3.8\,h$)

has been used for labor induction with a more favorable cervix is shown in Fig. 7.2 (Embrey *et al.*, 1980).

For induction of abortion a more prolonged duration of effect is required. The *in vitro* release from a pessary containing the analog 16,16-dimethyl *trans*-Δ_2 PGE_1 (ONO 802) with a half-life of 8 h is illustrated in Fig. 7.3; it has given promising results in the termination of early pregnancy.

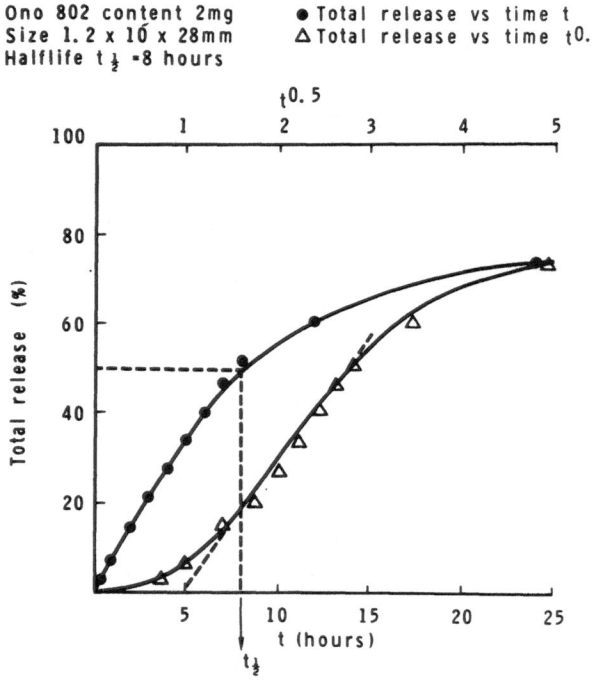

Figure 7.3 Release of ONO 802 from a dry PEO slice into buffer solution pH 7.4 at 37°C

STABILITY STUDIES

Pessaries were stored in plastic bags without exclusion of moisture or air, at room temperature or 4°C and representative pessaries from each batch formulated were assayed at intervals. A small sample (2–4 mg) was placed in 3 ml ethanol overnight. After shaking for 30 min the ethanol was removed, a further 3 ml ethanol added to the pessary and, after shaking for 15 min, the extracts combined, evaporated at 37°C under nitrogen and taken up in 10 ml phosphate buffer at pH 7.3.

PGE_2 content was assayed by radioimmunoassay using an antibody selective for PGE_2. Serial dilutions of the sample extract were prepared to provide an estimated working dilution of 1000 pg/ml and allow aliquots of 0.1 ml and 0.2 ml to fall within the range of the standard curve of the assay. PGE_2 standards were made from a stock solution to cover the range 20–1000 pg in 0.1 ml. 0.1 ml and 0.2 ml aliquots were assayed in triplicate, mean values calculated for each sample and by referring to the weight of the pessary, the total amount of PGE_2 remaining in the pessary was calculated.

The stability of PGE content in pessaries stored at 4 °C is shown in Table 7.1 and at room temperature in Table 7.2. Because the study of pessaries from different batches was commenced at different times the data available relate to six pessaries assayed at intervals up to 11–14 months, five pessaries at 9–10 months, up to 8 months in one other pessary, and 6 months or less in the remainder. Studied a shorter time, the data for stability at room temperature relate to one pessary at 12 months, two at 10 months and the remainder for 7 months or less.

No evidence of deterioration in the PGE_2 content of the pessaries at 4 °C was noted over an 11–14 month period. When the contents of the six pessaries in which data are available for up to 11–14 months was compared with the formulated content of the pessary, statistical analysis showed that there was no significant difference in the content ($p > 0.05$). Although the data are

Table 7.1 PGE_2 content (mg) of pessaries stored at 4°C

Formulated content	Months					
	1–2	*3–4*	*5–6*	*7–8*	*9–10*	*11–14*
10			·			10
10.4	11.11		10.6			
9.6	9.8	9.8	10.6		9.7	9.9
9.7	9.8		9.8		9.6	9.8
10	10					
9.7	10.6		9.3			
10	11.9					
9.9	11.0	11.0				
9.0	12.6					
15.0					15.8	15.8
15.8	16.9		16.8			
15.0	14.8	16.3		15.2		13.9
30.0						32.8

Table 7.2 PGE_2 content (mg) of pessaries stored at room temperature

Formulated content	Months					
	1–2	*3–4*	*5–6*	*7–8*	*9–10*	*11–12*
9.6		9.9	9.9		9.9	9.7
9.7	9.9		10.3		9.4	
9.7	10.0		9.7			
9.9		9.6				
15		15.2		15.3		

Table 7.3 Influence of initial cervical score on labor outcome following insertion of PGE$_2$

	Primigravidae cervical score			Multigravidae cervical score		
	0–3	4–5	6+	0–3	4–5	6+
Total No.	32	42	37	7	37	52
'Spontaneous' labor	20.9%	50.0%	56.8%	0%	48.6%	80.7%
Oxytocin	71.8%	35.7%	37.8%	42.8%	37.8%	11.5%
Epidural	50.0%	52.4%	24.5%	28.6%	24.3%	5.8%
Labor length (h)	10.6±5.2[1]	8.7±3.4[1]	7.3±4.0[1]	6.7±3.5[1]	5.2±1.8[1]	4.3±1.7[1]
Spontaneous vaginal delivery	34.3%	45.2%	62.2%	85.7%	94.5%	96.2%
Cesarean section	12.5%	9.5%	2.7%	14.3%	2.7%	0%
1-min Apgar score	8.5±0.6[1]	8.4±0.9[1]	8.5±1.1[1]	8.4±11[1]	8.5±0.7[1]	8.5±1.3[1]

[1] Mean ±SD

Table 7.4 Labor outcome related to labor establishment after PGE$_2$ polymer pessary alone

	0–3		4–5		6+	
	PGE established labor	PGE$_2$ + orthodox induction	PGE$_2$ established labor	PGE$_2$ + orthodox induction	PGE$_2$ established labor	PGE$_2$ + orthodox induction
No.	7	32	39	40	63	26
Epidural	28.5%	50.0%	33.3%	45.0%	3.2%	38.5%
Oxytocin	28.5%	75.0%	17.9%	55.0%	7.9%	65.4%
Spontaneous vaginal delivery	57.1%	40.6%	69.2%	67.5%	90.5%	61.5%
Cesarean section	0.0%	15.6%	2.6%	10.0%	0.0%	3.8%

fragmentary the evidence indicates that the PGE_2 content may be stable for a longer period than 12 months at 4 °C. While fewer studies have been carried out at room temperature, stability is evident for at least 6 months and probably longer.

The homogeneous distribution of PGE_2 in the pessary matrix was confirmed by comparing samples from opposite ends of the pessary. In eight tests there was no significant difference in PGE_2 content.

No attempt was made to seal stored pessaries. There is some evidence to suggest that deterioration of polymers can occur in the presence of extremes of moisture and oxygen over prolonged periods. Experiments are being undertaken to determine the extent to which exclusion of uncontrolled atmospheric conditions will extend long-term stability.

CLINICAL RESULTS

The clinical performance of a PGE_2-releasing pessary in labor induction in 207 patients is summarized in Tables 7.3 and 7.4. Labor was initiated by PG treatment alone in 20 % of primigravidae with an unripe cervix, while in multigravidae with a favorable cervix the need for orthodox labor induction was obviated in 80 % of patients. As the initial cervical score increased, so the labor prognosis improved; augmentation with oxytocin and epidural analgesia were less often required and spontaneous vaginal delivery was more common. Additionally, for each cervical score the clinical benefits were greatest when labour followed the PG treatment alone (Table 7.4). These results compare well with those reported using simple Witepsol PGE_2 pessaries.

In the induction of abortion preliminary trials have shown the clinical effectiveness of PGE analogs in a solitary polymer device. Thus in early post-conceptional pregnancy (menstrual induction), using 16,16-dimethyl *trans*-Δ_2 PGE_1 (ONO 802) complete abortion (i.e. negative pregnancy test, cessation of bleeding within 14 days), with few side effects, occurred in 27/32 women (84 %). An improved formulation compared with that first used resulted in success in 16/17 women (94 %). In second trimester women successful abortion (within 24 h) occurred in 12/14 (85 %).

Despite the clinical potential of vaginally administered prostaglandins in fertility regulation, attainment of the expected objectives has proved elusive because, in the products available hitherto, otherwise promising PGE analogs do not provide sustained release and lack long-term storage stability. The recent developments described demonstrate that these disadvantages can be overcome by improvements in the delivery vehicle.

References

Embrey, M. P., Graham, N. B. and McNeill, M. E. (1980). Induction of labour with a sustained-release prostaglandin E₂ vaginal pessary. *Br. Med. J.*, **281**, 901–5

Hendricks, C. H., Dingfelder, J. R. and Gruber, W. S. (1976). Clinical observations with a prostaglandin-containing silastic vaginal device for pregnancy termination. *Prostaglandins*, **12**, Suppl., 99–122

Lauerson, N. H. and Wilson, K. H. (1976). The abortifacient effectiveness and plasma prostaglandin concentrations with 15(S)-15-methyl prostaglandin F_2 methyl ester-containing vaginal silastic devices. *Fertil. Steril.,* **27**, 1366–73

Tejuja, S., Choudhury, S. D., Manchanda, P. K. and Malhotra, U. (1979). Indian experience with a single long-acting vaginal suppository for the termination of pregnancies. *Contraception,* **19**, 191–6

8
Laminaria Treatment prior to Late Mid-trimester Abortion by Uterine Evacuation

P. G. STUBBLEFIELD, A. M. ALTMAN and S. P. GOLDSTEIN

INTRODUCTION

Dilatation and evacuation (D&E) has increasingly been recognized as an important alternative when abortion is required in the mid-trimester (Grimes *et al.*, 1977; Cates, 1979). There is as yet no consensus as to the details of the procedure. Peterson (1979) has advocated forcible cervical dilatation with large metal dilators. Hanson (1978) and Barr (1978) have used laminaria tents left in place overnight prior to evacuation. Bierer and Steiner (1971) used forcible dilatation plus successive sets of laminaria replaced every few hours over a 40-h period. Our own experience with D&E at 13–16½ weeks convinced us of the desirability of at least overnight placement of laminaria (Altman *et al.*, 1981). We wished to extend our range for D&E still further into the mid-trimester, but we were concerned about possible operative difficulty and excessive blood loss. Accordingly, we performed a randomized trial of two different protocols for laminaria treatment prior to late mid-trimester D&E.

METHODOLOGY

Sixty women who requested abortion at 17–19 menstrual weeks volunteered for the randomized study and gave written informed consent. Ultrasound measurement of fetal size was used frequently to confirm that gestational age was less than 20 weeks. Allocation to treatment Group A or B was determined in order of entry into the study using a list generated from a table of random numbers. Group A received one set of three to seven small or medium laminaria japonicum tents (purchased from Medispec, 3483 Golden Gate Way, PO Box 53, Lafayette, California 94549) and the abortions were performed the next morning, 18–22 h after laminaria placement. Group B patients returned on the second day for removal of the first set of laminaria and insertion of a second set of 7–19 tents. Their abortions were performed on the third day, 44–48 h after the first insertion of laminaria. Prior to laminaria insertion the upper vagina and cervix were cleansed with povidone iodide and the cervix was grasped with a tenaculum. Laminaria were inserted one at a time into the cervical canal until the upper end was just above the internal os. After all laminaria were in place, two 4×4 gauze sponges were packed over the cervix and into the fornices to prevent expulsion.

Both patient groups returned to their homes after laminaria placement. All were given acetaminophen to take as needed for pain, and all were advised to take oral tetracycline 500 mg four times a day from laminaria insertion until 24 h after the abortion.

Cervical calibration

The internal diameter of the cervical canal was determined three times: (1) prior to laminaria placement, (2) immediately prior to the abortion, and (3) at the follow-up visit 2 weeks post-abortally. The largest Hegar dilator that passed the internal cervical os without resistance was taken as the calibration.

Pain from laminaria

All patients were questioned just prior to the abortion as to the amount of discomfort caused by laminaria treatment. This was recorded on a 5-point scale ranging from none to severe enough to prevent sleep or to produce vomiting.

The abortion procedure

After laminaria removal the upper vagina was cleansed with povidone iodide and paracervical block was established. We used lidocaine 0.5% with epinephrine 1 : 200 000 because epinephrine has been reported to reduce operative blood loss (Hanson, 1978). Twenty cubic centimeters was injected deeply into the cervical stroma at multiple injection sites as described by Finks (1973). Fentanyl 0.05 mg and diazepam 5 mg, were given slowly into a running intravenous line for additional analgesia and sedation. General anesthesia was never used. We waited 3 min for the full effect of the paracervical block, and then ruptured the fetal membranes by inserting a 16 mm vacuum cannula into the uterine cavity and turning on the suction for a few seconds. The amniotic fluid was drained through the cannula and discarded. The surgeon then used the 16 mm cannula and large-bore vacuum system (purchased from Rocket of London, Inc., PO Box 407, Branford, Connecticut 06405, or Medispec) in alternation with a Sopher forcep to evacuate the uterus. The procedures were performed in a treatment room of our hospital abortion unit.

Operating time

Timing of the procedure was started when the surgeon began uterine evacuation after the amniotic fluid had been drained. Timing was stopped when the surgeon judged the uterus empty and laid down his instruments for the last time.

Measured blood loss

After discarding the amniotic fluid, all fluid issuing from the vagina was collected either in the vacuum bottle, or in a basin at the patient's buttocks. After the procedure a measured 300 cm³ of water was aspirated through the vacuum cannula, the gauze specimen bag was manually compressed, and the 300 cm³ deducted from the total.

Post-abortal care and follow-up

Patients were observed for 2 h post-procedure, instructed about contraception and self-care, and discharged. They were given a 24 h phone number for emergency use and a questionnaire to return by mail. All were asked to return for a 2-week post-abortal visit, but many preferred to return to their referring physicians. Three months after completion of study an additional brief questionnaire was mailed to all subjects in an additional effort to discover complications.

Gestational age

Final gestational age was determined post-procedure by measurement of the fetal foot length as reported by Streeter (1920).

RESULTS

Patient characteristics

Mean age of Group A patients was 21.1 ± 5.1 years, standard deviation, and did not differ from the mean age of Group B patients, 22.6 ± 5.6 years. Group A did contain more primigravid women than Group B ($\chi^2 = 4.3$; $p = 0.039$) as shown in Table 8.1. Thirty percent of the total sample reported at least one previous induced abortion. Mean cervical calibrations prior to laminaria

Table 8.1 Previous obstetric history

	Group A	Group B
Gravida 1, para. 0	15	6
Gravida 2, para. 1	4	4
Gravida 2, induced abortion 1	8	5
Gravida 3 or more	5	13
One or more induced abortions	9	11

Gravida 1, para. 0 vs. all others, $\chi^2 = 4.3$; $p = 0.039$

placement did not differ: Group A was 7.0 ± 1.5 mm and Group B was 6.9 ± 1.4 mm.

Relevant medical history was present in two cases in Group A: previous pelvic inflammatory disease and an active scabies infestation. In Group B one patient had asthma, one had neurofibromatosis, one had rheumatoid arthritis, and one had a positive cervical culture for gonorrhea necessitating antibiotic treatment before laminaria could be inserted.

Results of laminaria treatment

Considerable cervical dilatation was accomplished by the laminaria treatment in both study groups (Table 8.2). Greater post-treatment dilatation and a greater difference between pre- and post-treatment calibrations was accomplished by the 2-day regimen, Group B, than by the 1-day regimen, Group A. Equivalent post-treatment dilatations and dilatation differences were seen for nulliparous and parous women.

Unfortunately, more patients in Group B reported pain during laminaria treatment (Table 8.3). Rupture of the fetal membranes during laminaria

Table 8.2 Cervical calibrations before and after laminaria treatment

| Parity | Group | N | Cervical calibrations, Mean $\pm$ SD (mm) | | |
			Pre-treatment	Post-treatment	Change in dilatation
Para. 0	A	24	6.8 ± 1.6	18.0 ± 2.7^1	11.3 ± 2.5^4
	B	12	6.3 ± 0.8	22.8 ± 2.8	16.4 ± 3.1
Para. 1	A	8	7.6 ± 0.9	18.7 ± 1.4^2	11.0 ± 1.2^5
	B	16	7.3 ± 1.7	22.1 ± 3.2	14.8 ± 2.9
Total	A	32	7.0 ± 1.5	18.2 ± 2.4^3	11.2 ± 2.2^6
	B	28	6.9 ± 1.4	22.4 ± 3.0	15.5 ± 3.0

Group A compared to Group B by Student's t-test
[1] $T = 4.97; p < 0.01$
[2] $T = 2.85; p < 0.01$
[3] $T = 6.02; p < 0.01$
[4] $T = 5.32; p < 0.01$
[5] $T = 3.53; p < 0.01$
[6] $T = 6.38; p < 0.01$

Table 8.3 Pain reported during laminaria treatment

Patient report	Group A	Group B
No pain	12	3
Mild pain	8	15
Moderate pain	7	5
Severe pain, able to sleep	1	2
Severe pain, not able to sleep	3	3
Not stated	1	0

No pain $vs.$ all others, $\chi^2 = 5.7; p = 0.017$

treatment occurred in four cases in Group A and in three cases in Group B. In one of the Group B cases the membranes ruptured prior to placement of the second set of laminaria and the abortion was done at 18 h. In another Group B case the membranes prolapsed through a widely dilated cervix when the first set of laminaria were removed. Her abortion was performed immediately. Both cases were left in Group B for analysis although they did not receive 2 days of laminaria treatment.

Uterine evacuation

The surgeons experienced difficulty in extracting the fetal calvarium in six Group A cases and in only two Group B cases, but these frequencies were not statistically separable. One of these Group A cases required a second uterine evacuation procedure which was carried out 2 h after the first. By then the retained calvarium had been pushed into the lower uterine segment by uterine contractions and was readily retrieved without resort to general anesthesia. This case was the only immediate complication in the series. The surgeons reported the procedure as 'easy' in seven Group A cases and in 14 Group B cases ($\chi^2 = 5.2$; $p = 0.023$), supporting the notion that the greater cervical dilatation accomplished by 2 days of laminaria did facilitate the uterine evacuation.

Operating time

There were no important differences in operating time between the two groups when compared by one-way analysis of variance (ANOVA) or by Student's t-test between individual gestational age groupings (Table 8.4). The few cases at 19 weeks in Group B went faster than those of comparable gestational age in Group A; however, the numbers of cases are too few to support generalization. Only three cases in each group required 10 min or longer for uterine evacuation (Group A, 10.3, 15.8 and 21.4 min; Group B, 10.0, 11.6 and 15.3 min).

Table 8.4 Operating time

Gestational age[1] (weeks)	Group A		Group B	
	N	Mean ± SD (min)	N	Mean ± SD (min)
14	0	—	1	2.7
15	1	4.6	0	—
16	6	4.3 ± 1.4	2	5.2 ± 1.6
17	8	5.9 ± 2.2	9	6.6 ± 3.8
18	15	7.4 ± 4.2	12	6.4 ± 1.7
19	2	11.6 ± 6.0	3	5.5 ± 2.4
20	0	—	1	11.6
Total	32	6.6 ± 3.7	28	6.3 ± 2.7
17 and over	25	7.0 ± 4.2	25	6.6 ± 2.8

[1] As determined post-abortally by measurement of fetal foot length (Johnstone et al., 1976)

Measured blood loss

Comparison of Groups A and B as to blood loss revealed no important differences by ANOVA or by Student's t-test, although, as in the case of operating time, the few cases done after 18 weeks did suggest some advantage for Group B (Table 8.5). Blood loss never exceeded 450 cm^3 and in no case was transfusion required.

One surgeon performed 18 of Group A cases and 15 of Group B. A second surgeon did nine of Group A and seven of Group B, while a third surgeon did five cases in Group A and six in Group B. All three have had extensive experience with mid-trimester D&E, and neither operating time nor blood loss differed significantly between surgeons.

Complications

The only immediate complication was the Group A case previously described where a second uterine evacuation procedure was needed prior to discharge. The rate for total immediate complications is thus 1 in 60 or 1.7 %. There were no cervical lacerations, no perforations and no major surgical procedures needed to treat complications. Late complications, occurring after discharge, were reported by four patients, a rate for late complications of 6.7 %. One Group A patient had a uterine curettage for bleeding 3 weeks post-abortally. Her 2-week examination had been normal. A Group B patient reported fever to 101°F (38.3°C) during the first 24 h after abortion. This resolved without treatment. Neither patient had taken the prescribed tetracycline. One Group A patient reported treatment for vaginitis and vaginal bleeding that lasted for 28 days post-procedure. Another Group A patient reported a transient dysuria with negative urine culture. Follow-up information was obtained for 17 Group A patients (53.1 %) and for 17 Group B patients (60.7 %). The rate of total late complications for patients with follow-up was thus 11.8 %. However, none of our complications would be considered major complications by the Center for Disease Control Criteria (Peterson, 1979).

Table 8.5 Measured blood loss

Gestational age[1] (weeks)	Group A		Group B	
	N	Mean ± SD (cm^3)	N	Mean ± SD (cm^3)
14	0	—	1	50.0
15	1	40.0	0	—
16	6	86.7 ± 53.1	2	85.0 ± 35.4
17	8	210.6 ± 135.3	9	109.4 ± 95.6
18	15	189.3 ± 98.2	12	197.5 ± 106.1
19	2	260.0 ± 84.9	3	121.7 ± 20.2
20	0	—	1	110.0
Total	32	175.2 ± 110.3	28	144.6 ± 98.7
17 and over	25	201.0 ± 108.0	25	153.2 ± 100.7

[1] As determined post-abortally by measurement of fetal foot length (Johnstone et al., 1976)

The post-abortal cervix

The cervical canal was recalibrated 2 weeks post-abortally for ten cases in Group A and seven in Group B. Mean internal diameter of the cervical canal in the Group A patients was 3.9 ± 1.4 mm and 2.9 ± 1.2 mm in Group B; means that are not statistically separable. In every case where post-abortal calibration was performed, the diameter was less than it had been prior to laminaria placement.

Two days of laminaria treatment did confer any benefit: uterine evacuation was made easier as judged by the surgeons, and there were fewer cases where difficulty was encountered in removing all of the fetal tissue. We were unable to show any important difference in blood loss or operating time. As it turned out, most of our cases were at 17 or 18 menstrual weeks. Had more been of later gestational ages, the suggestion of reduction of blood loss and operating time in Group B might have been confirmed. The 2 days of laminaria treatment produced more patient discomfort, added another patient visit, and additional expense of lodging and food for out-of-town patients. We conclude that for patients at 18 weeks or less, the benefits of 2 days laminaria treatment are not sufficient to offset the added cost in pain and expense for the patient.

We did not implement the protocol of Hern and Oakes (1977) which makes use of four sets of laminaria rather than two because of logistic difficulties and the greater expense of still more laminaria. Such a protocol with resultant greater cervical dilatation might be important if D&E were performed at gestational ages 19 weeks and beyond.

As American practitioners have begun to do more mid-trimester abortions at advanced gestational ages by D&E procedures, the benefit of 2 days treatment has become more apparent. Darney has reported using 2 days of laminaria in procedures done as late as 22–23 weeks, and feels strongly that this treatment plan reduces the risk of perforation and allows obstetricians and gynecologists in training to do these more difficult procedures with ease (Darney, 1983).

Our post-abortal cervical calibrations showed recovery of the cervical canal to a small diameter, and therefore differ from the findings of Johnstone *et al.* (1976). They found that forcible dilatation of the cervix beyond 11 mm was associated with a long-lasting increase in the diameter of the canal. Our work suggests that the more gentle and prolonged dilatation produced by laminaria tents is more completely reversible than is forcible dilatation with a metal dilator. If, as has been suggested, forcible dilatation to larger diameters may endanger later desired pregnancy (Stubblefield *et al.*, 1978), laminaria tents may be preferred for cervical dilatation prior to mid-trimester D&E.

CONCLUDING REMARKS

Our routine procedure for early mid-trimester abortion is laminaria dilatation of the cervix followed the next day by instrumental evacuation of the uterus. In order to determine whether an additional day of laminaria treatment would facilitate later mid-trimester abortion procedures, we carried out a randomized trial of two laminaria regimens. Group A patients had laminaria tents placed in the cervical canal for 18–22 h prior to uterine evacuation with a large-bore vacuum cannula system and Sopher forceps (D&E). Group B patients had a second set of laminaria placed after removal of the first, and laminaria treatment for a total of 44–48 h prior to evacuation. Calibrations of the cervical canals after laminaria treatment were significantly greater for Group B (22.4 ± 3.0 mm) than for Group A (18.2 ± 2.4 mm). There were somewhat fewer difficult procedures in Group B, and the surgeons more often rated Group B cases as 'easy'; however, operative time and measured blood loss did not differ for the two groups. Immediate and late complications were minimal. Cervical calibrations 2 weeks post-abortally showed recovery of the cervices to diameters smaller than those measured before laminaria placement.

References

Altman, A. M., Stubblefield, P. G., Parker, K., Winger, D. and Osathanondh, R. (1981). Midtrimester abortion by laminaria and vacuum evacuation (L&E) on a teaching service: a review of 789 cases. *Adv. Plann. Parent.*, **16**, 1–6

Barr, M. M. (1978). Midtrimester abortion at 12 to 20 weeks by dilatation and evacuation method under local anesthesia. *Adv. Plann. Parent.*, **13**, 16–20

Bierer, I. and Steiner, V. (1971). Termination of pregnancy in the second trimester with the aid of laminaria tents. *Med. Gynecol. Sociol.*, **6**, 9–10

Cates, W., Jr. (1979). D&E after 12 weeks: safe or hazardous? *Contemp. Obstet. Gynecol.*, **13**, 23–30

Darney, P. D. (1983). Midtrimester abortion under ultrasound Guidance. Postgraduate Course. (Tampa, Florida: National Abortion Federation, 31 January)

Finks, A. I. (1973). Midtrimester abortion. *Lancet*, **1**, 263–4

Grimes, D. A., Schulz, K. F., Cates, W., Jr. *et al.* (1977). Midtrimester abortion by dilatation and evacuation. A safe and practical alternative. *N. Engl. J. Med.*, **296**, 1141–5

Grimes, D. A., Schulz, K. F., Cates, W., Jr. and Tyler, C. W., Jr. (1979). Local versus general anesthesia: Which is safer for performing suction curettage abortion? *Am. J. Obstet. Gynecol.*, **135**, 1030–5

Hanson, M. S. (1978). D&E midtrimester abortion preceeded by laminaria. Paper presented at the Sixteenth Annual Meeting of the Association of Planned Parenthood Physicians, San Diego, California, 26 October

Hern, W. M. and Oakes, A. G. (1977). Multiple laminaria treatment in early midtrimester outpatient suction abortion: a preliminary report. *Adv. Plann. Parent.*, **12**, 93–7

Johnstone, F. D., Beard, R. J., Boyd, I. E. and McCarthy, T. G. (1976). Cervical diameter after suction termination of pregnancy. *Br. Med. J.*, **1**, 68–9

Peterson, W. (1979). Dilatation and evacuation. Patient evaluation and surgical techniques. In Zatuchni, G. I., Sciarra, J. J. and Spiedel, J. J. (eds.) *Pregnancy Termination: Procedures, Safety, and New Developments*. pp. 184–190. (Hagerstown: Harper & Row)

Streeter, G. L. (1920). Weight, sitting height, head size, foot length and menstrual age of the human embryo. *Contrib. Embryol. Carnegie*, **11**, 157–67

Stubblefield, P. G., Albrecht, B. H., Koos, B. and Fredericksen, M. (1978). A randomized study of 12 mm. and 15.9 mm. cannulas in midtrimester abortion by laminaria and vacuum curettage. *Fertil. Steril.*, **29**, 512–17

Wright, C. S. W., Campbell, S. and Beazley, J. (1972). Second trimester abortion after vaginal termination of pregnancy. *Lancet*, **1**, 1278–9

9
Ethacridine (Rivanol ®)–catheter technique in second trimester abortion

C. A. INGEMANSON

At present the mortality and morbidity is higher in mid-trimester than in first trimester abortion, and even if the mid-trimester abortions are few in many countries, there is a need to find safe and effective methods to interrupt a mid-trimester pregnancy. Since the early 1960s the most frequently used method for second trimester abortion in Sweden has been the intra- or extra-amniotic instillation of 20 % saline. A report by Bengtsson in 1967 of three deaths and a number of serious complications in 6161 saline abortions prompted investigation of other and safer methods. The saline method has gradually been abandoned, and is mainly used in the few pregnancies which are interrupted after the 20th week of gestation as the saline method causes fetal death which is not achieved with prostaglandins or ethacridine–catheter in most cases. Prostaglandins, or the ethacridine–catheter method, are nowadays the most commonly used ways to interrupt a mid-trimester pregnancy in Sweden.

ETHACRIDINE LACTATE (RIVANOL)

Ethacridine lactate (Rivanol) (6,9-diamino-2-oxyethyl acridine lactate) is a yellow dye with antiseptic properties. It was first prepared by Roser and Jensch in 1920 and has been used mainly as a skin disinfectant and for wound treatment but also intra-abdominally after intestinal surgery and orally against diarrhea. The toxicity in studies in mice and rabbits is low ($LD_{50} = 50-120$ mg/kg) but modern toxicological studies on man are lacking. We know, however, that large volumes of 0.1 % ethacridine lactate can be nephrotoxic. Pytel et al. (1963) in the Soviet Union have reported five cases of acute renal insufficiency, four of which were of a temporary nature with the use of 500–700 ml 0.1 % ethacridine lactate. Thus it is important to consider that any solution deposited in the uterus can be absorbed rapidly into the systemic circulation. For this reason the solution chosen for intrauterine infusion should be as safe to the woman as if the same amount of solution were injected intravenously. Moderate amounts of 0.1 % ethacridine lactate up to a maximum of 200 ml can be used, as it is safe to the patient and has the advantage of being antiseptic. Extra-amniotic instillation of ethacridine lactate was first used for abortion by Kashiwara and Fujibayashi (1949) in Japan using 30–200 ml 0.1 % Rivanol® (Farbwerke Hoechst AG, Frankfurt, West Germany), ethacridine lactate, and the method has been used extensively in Japan for the last 30 years without any known serious side effects.

Early studies by Sepeika (1934) have shown that ethacridine lactate has a slight oxytocic effect but this is most probably unimportant for the abortifacient effect. Studies by Gustavii (1977) suggest that the abortifacient effect of ethacridine lactate is due to prostaglandin synthesis in the decidual cells. Support for this mode of action is given by Ölund (1981), who has shown that the amniotic fluid levels of prostaglandin E_2, prostaglandin $F_{2\alpha}$ thromboxane B2 and 6-keto-PGF$_{2\alpha}$ increased after induction with ethacridin lactate. There was also increase in the amniotic fluid of the prostaglandin and thromboxane precursor arachidonic acid. Ölund (1979) has also shown that indomethacin, a strong prostaglandin synthetase inhibitor, significantly prolonged the instillation–abortion period in ethacridine lactate-induced abortions.

The effect of ethacridine lactate on the coagulation system has also been studied by Ölund (1981) with special reference to disseminated intravascular coagulation. A low-level activation of the coagulation system was found, but this was of the same magnitude as in a control group of women with spontaneous abortion. There is no indication that ethacridine lactate can provoke disseminated intravascular coagulation that has been reported in saline- and urea-induced abortions. Data collected from eight gynecological departments in Sweden in 2058 consecutive ethacridine lactate mid-trimester abortions did not show any fatal or life-threatening complication (Ingemanson, 1979). The only major complications encountered were one case of cervical fistula in a young nulliparous woman with a rigid cervix, and one case of deep cervical tear. Thus I believe we can state that the extra-amniotic ethacridine–catheter method is a safe procedure when moderate doses of a 0.1 % solution are given.

Ingemanson (1973) compared 0.1 % ethacridine lactate extra-amniotically and 20 % saline extra-amniotically for mid-trimester abortion in 106 consecutive cases. Alternating patients were administered either 20 % saline extra-amniotically or 0.1 % ethacridine lactate extra-amniotically followed by insertion of a catheter (a Nelaton no. 16) into the uterine cavity until only 1–2 cm protruded from the cervix; this was left in place until abortion occurred. In the saline cases the catheter was withdrawn directly after instillation. The induction–abortion intervals in the two groups were similar but there was a considerable difference in side effects even if no serious complications occurred.

The amount of solution used in both groups was 10 ml per week of pregnancy up to a maximum of 150 ml. No oxytocin was used in this study. In the saline group 12 experienced considerable pain and four slight pain. Four experienced nausea and vomiting, three a sudden temporary fall in blood pressure and four a sensation of overall warmth. Side effects in the ethacridine–catheter group were limited to one case of slight pain during instillation. Signs of infection were more common in the saline group. Sixteen patients had a 1-day temperature rise of 38 °C or more compared to five in the ethacridine–catheter group. Seven patients in the saline group and two in the ethacridine–catheter group were in fever for 2 days or more. Two patients in the saline group, and one patient in the ethacridine–catheter group, developed post-abortion salpingitis within 1 month.

Himmelman *et al.* (1975) studied 302 consecutive cases of extra-amniotic saline abortions, 200 consecutive cases of extra-amniotic ethacridine–catheter abortions and 50 consecutive cases with extra-amniotic $PGF_{2\alpha}$. The criteria for complications were the same in the three groups. The catheter technique in the ethacridine–catheter cases was different from ours. A Foley catheter with a $10 \, cm^3$ balloon was used and left in place for 24 h. Bleeding, suspected infection and manifest infection were more frequent in the saline and $PGF_{2\alpha}$ groups.

The ethacridine–catheter group had a total complication rate of 10.5 % compared to 22 % with $PGF_{2\alpha}$ and 29 % with 20 % extra-aminotic saline. Besides a low complication rate another requirement of a good method of second trimester abortion is a high success rate within a reasonable period of time. The ethacridine–catheter method has shown a high success rate within 48–72 h of instillation. In different studies the abortion rate is 28–52 % within 24 h, 79–100 % within 48 h, and 88–100 % within 72 h.

Fylling and Refsdal (1973) tested different catheter techniques and obtained the fastest induction–abortion time when using a Foley catheter. In the ethacridine–catheter study with the best results, 100 % abortions within 48 h, a Foley catheter with a large $30 \, cm^3$ balloon was used (Ölund, 1979). At present, one of the most popular methods in Japan for mid-trimester abortions is the use of a laminaria tent in the cervical canal followed by a metreurynter, a cone-shaped balloon, in the lower uterine segment and this metreurynter is given a mechanical stretch. By using a Foley catheter with a large balloon one will likely create a metreurynter effect and thereby speed up the abortion process. Recent studies by Manabe *et al.* (1982) indicate that the effect caused by metreurynter or catheters in the uterine cavity is at least partly mediated through the synthesis of prostaglandins.

RECOMMENDED TECHNIQUE

For the last 2 years we have used the following technique:

(1) Thorough cleansing of the vagina with an antiseptic solution (0.05 % chlorhexidine).
(2) A Foley catheter no. 18 with a $30 \, cm^3$ balloon filled with 0.1 % ethacridine lactate (Rivanol) is introduced via the cervical canal just past the internal os.
(3) The catheter balloon is filled with $30 \, cm^3$ physiological saline.
(4) Aspiration check for blood. If clear blood flows into catheter or syringe as aspiration, a new attempt is made after 2 h.
(5) If no blood flows into the catheter or syringe $150 \, cm^3$ (irrespective of the

week of pregnancy) of a 0.1 % solution of Rivanol is gently instilled in the extraovular space in 3–4 min.

(6) The catheter is fixed to the thigh with a slight stretch.

(7) The catheter is left in place for 24 h (if the patient is not aborting earlier).

(8) If the abortion has not started within 20 h an intravenous infusion of oxytocin is started (70 IU in 1000 cm³ 5.5 % glucose) and repeated every 12th hour until abortion occurs.

(9) If no abortion has occurred within 48 h the above procedure is repeated.

RECENT DATA

The present study group of 43 consecutive cases represents all late legal abortions carried out at the clinic in the 2-year period June 1980 to July 1982. The distribution according to completed pregnancy weeks is shown in Fig. 9.1. The assessment of the gestational age was made according to the last menstrual period and clinical examination. If there was any doubt about the length of gestation an ultrasound examination was performed. The instillations were carried out by experienced, as well as less experienced, doctors of the staff. There were no complications in conjunction with the ethacridine–catheter procedure, only a slight backward leakage of ethacridine lactate in one case. In

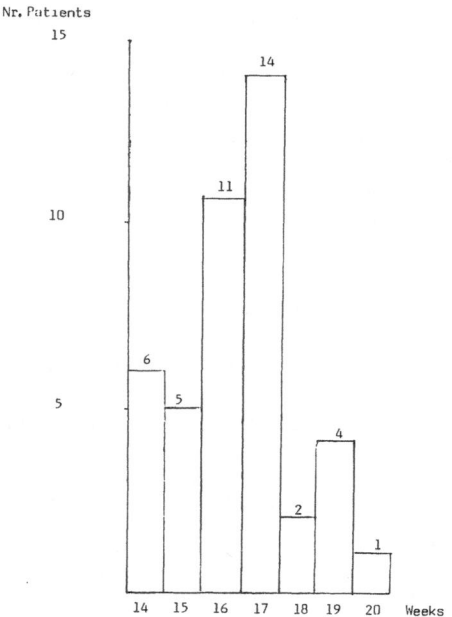

Figure 9.1 Completed pregnancy weeks (43 patients)

86

none of the cases had the procedure to be postponed due to blood at the aspiration check before the instillation. Nine patients aborted within 24 h, 23 within 36 h and 11 within 48 h. This means a cumulative abortion rate of 20 % at 24 h, 72 % at 36 h and 98 % at 48 h (Fig. 9.2). The mean instillation–abortion time in the successful cases (abortion within 48 h) was 31 h with a range of 10–48 h. Only one patient failed to abort within 48 h, and was reinstilled and aborted 85 h after the first instillation. In all cases where it was not obvious that the patient had aborted completely, a curettage was performed immediately after the abortion. All patients were treated in the hospital and stayed for 2 days after the abortion took place.

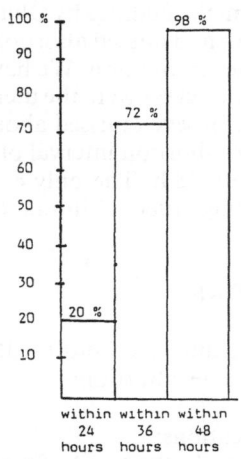

Figure 9.2 Cumulative abortion rate (43 patients)

SIDE EFFECTS AND COMPLICATIONS

Side effects and complications are shown in Table 9.1. One case of deep cervical tear occurred in a young nulliparous woman with a rigid cervix. The tear healed well after primary suturing. Five patients had a 1-day temperature

Table 9.1 Side effects and complications (43 cases)

Fever ≥ 38 °C 1 day	5
Fever ≥ 38 °C 2 days or more	0
Salpingitis post ab.	1
Cervical tear	1
Blood loss more than	1
500 ml	1
1000 ml	1
Blood transfusion	0

rise of 38 °C or more. No antibiotics were given in these cases and none of the patients developed signs of a post-operative salpingitis. No patient was in fever for more than 1 day. One patient developed a laparoscopically verified salpingitis 14 days post-abortion. Excessive bleeding was uncommon but the bleeding was measured to 1200 ml in one case and 800 ml in another case. In no case was blood transfusion found necessary.

ETHACRIDINE–CATHETER IN FETAL DEATH, MISSED AND MOLAR PREGNANCY

We have been able to confirm the findings by Ölund (1981) that the method can be used in cases of fetal death and missed abortion. In three cases of fetal death all delivered within 22 h after instillation. We have used the method in missed abortion and molar pregnancy cases were the uterine size exceeded the size of a normal 12 weeks gestation. In seven missed abortion cases all aborted within 36 h with a mean induction–abortion interval of 25 h. In three cases of molar pregnancy all aborted within 48 h. The only complication encountered was one case of excessive bleeding; 1000 ml in one of the missed abortion cases.

CONCLUDING REMARKS

The extra-amniotic ethacridine (Rivanol)–catheter method offers many advantages in second trimester abortion:

(1)   no known contraindications;
(2)   safe to the patient, even in the hand of less experienced doctors, in the recommended doses and concentrations;
(3)   easy, usually painless, once-only procedure;
(4)   low complication rate;
(5)   high success rate within 48 h;
(6)   inexpensive;
(7)   can be used successfully also in cases of intrauterine fetal death, missed abortion and molar pregnancy.

The disadvantage is that the method does not generally cause fetal death, and it is not recommended to exceed the 20th week of pregnancy.

References

Bengtsson, L. P. (1967). Legal abortion by intrauterine injections. *Läkartidningen*, **64**, 5037
Fylling, P. and Refsdal, A. (1973). Rivanol induced midtrimester abortion. *Arch. Gynaecol.*, **215**, 359
Gustavii, B. (1977). Rivanol induced alterations of cultured cells. *Contraception*, **1**, 89
Himmelman, A., Myhrman, P. and Svanberg, S. G. (1975). Induction of second trimester abortion. Comparison between Rivanol and prostaglandin F_2-alfa regarding time factors and complications. *Contraception*, **12**, 645

Ingemanson, C. A. (1973). Legal abortion by extra-amniotic instillation of Rivanol in combination with rubber catheter insertion into the uterus after the twelfth week of pregnancy. *Am. J. Obstet. Gynecol.*, **115**, 211

Ingemanson, C. A. (1979). The ethacridine–catheter method in second-trimester abortion. In Zatuchni, G. I., Sciarra, J. J. and Speidel, J. J. (eds) *Pregnancy Termination, Procedures, Safety and New Developments.* p. 277. (Hagerstown: Harper & Row)

Kashiwara, N. and Fujibayashi, Y. (1949). Interruption of pregnancy by extraovular instillation of a solution. *Sanfu, Shinpo*, **1**, 24

Manabe, Y., Manabe, A. and Sagawa, N. (1982). Stretch-induced cervical softening and initiation of labor at term. *Acta Obstet. Gynecol. Scand.*, **61**, 279

Ölund, A. R. (1979). The effect of indomethacin on the instillation–abortion interval in Rivanol induced midtrimester abortion. *Acta Obstet. Gynecol. Scand.*, **58**, 121

Ölund, A. R. (1981). Extra-amniotic instillation of Rivanol in the management of patients with missed abortion and fetal death. *Acta Obstet. Gynecol. Scand.*, **60**, 313

Ölund, A. R. and Bistoletti, P. (1980). Koagulations und fibrinolysesystem bei Rivanol induzierten schwangershaftsabbruch. *Zbl. Gynäkol.*, **102**, 507

Ölund, A. R. and Larsson, B. (1978). Comparison of extraamniotic instillation of Rivanol and PGF$_2$-alfa either separately or in combination followed by oxytocin for second trimester abortion. *Acta Obstet. Gynecol. Scand.,* **57**, 333

Ölund, A. R., Kindahl, H., Oliw, E., Lindgren, J. Ā. and Larsson, B. (1980). Prostaglandins and thromboxanes in amniotic fluid during Rivanol-induced abortion and labour. *Prostaglandins*, **19** (15), 791

Pytel, A. Y., Lopatkin, N. A. and Kuchinsky, I. N. (1963). Acute renal insufficiency associated with intrauterine retromembranous administration of Rivanol for the interruption of pregnancy and its treatment with hemodialysis. *Akush. Ginek. (MoSk).*, **39**, 5

Sepeika, N. (1934). The action of acriflavine on the uterus. *J. Pharm. Pharmacol.*, **7**, 44

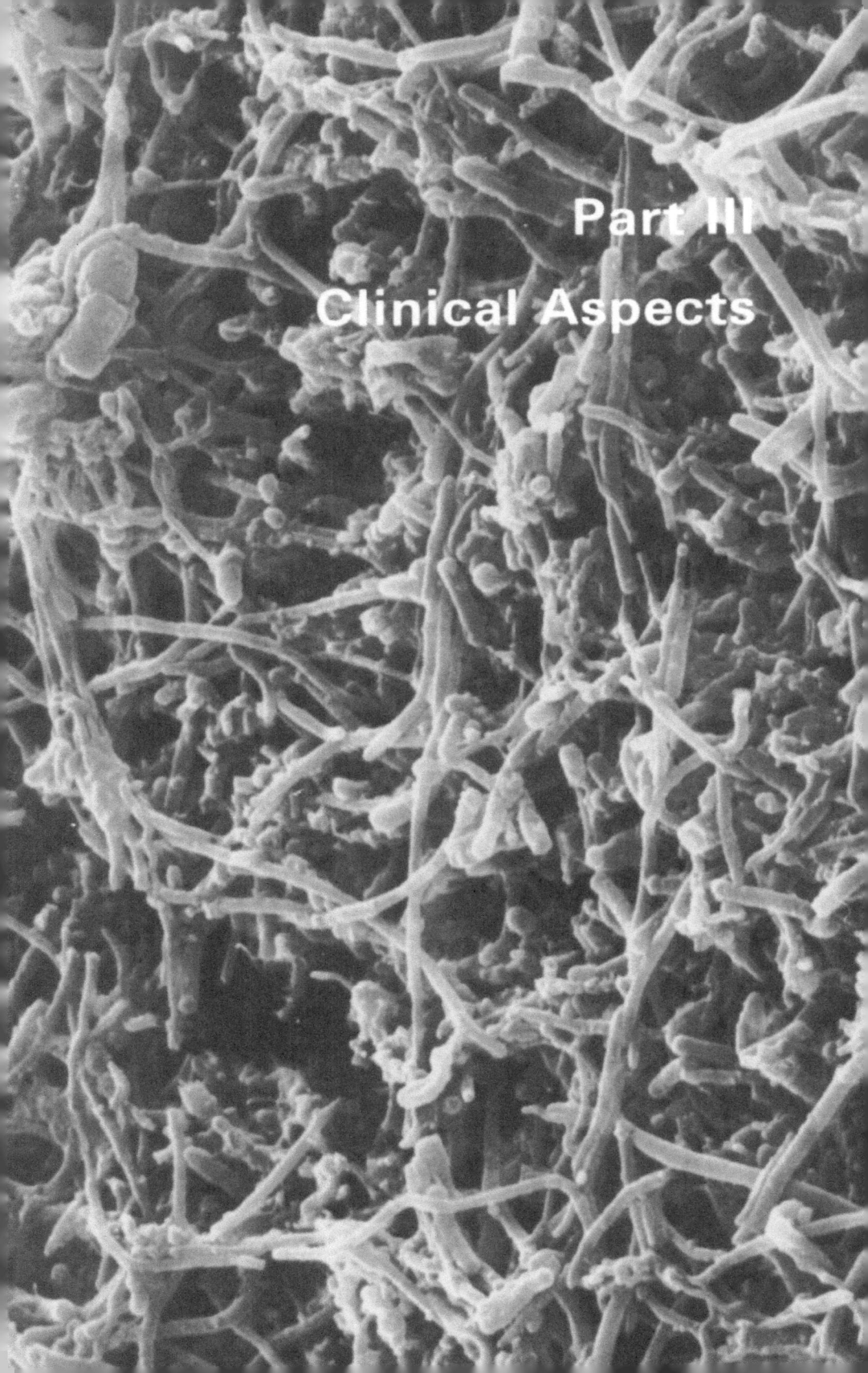

Part III
Clinical Aspects

10
Hemostasis in abortion

R. C. BRIEL

Hemostatic disorders in abortion are rare. However, when they occur they can lead to serious complications. Abortion curettage in the first trimester has a hemorrhage rate of 0.06 % (Grimes and Cates, 1979). Increased blood loss is usually due to incomplete abortion, laceration, perforation or uterine atony rather than coagulation disorders (Moberg *et al.*, 1975). Severe hemorrhage in itself can induce consumptive coagulopathy. No case of amniotic fluid embolism (AFE) in the first trimester of pregnancy has been reported so far (Guidotti *et al.*, 1981).

The risk of hemostatic disorders increases as pregnancy progresses and is most marked in pathological pregnancy. In the second trimester hemorrhage and transfusion rates vary from 2 to 8 % and 0.2 to 1.5 % respectively depending on duration of gestation and the methods used (Harman *et al.*, 1981; Grimes and Cates, 1979). In 26 % fatal embolism, mainly AFE with disseminated intravascular coagulation (DIC), was the cause of death associated in legal abortion induced by different methods, in the USA from 1972 to 1978 (Guidotti *et al.*, 1981). AFE can occur in patients with missed abortion or late therapeutic abortion, who have vigorous labor as a result of pharmacological stimulation (Bonnar, 1981). DIC and/or AFE may also be observed after dilatation and evacuation (Koplik, 1977; Strome and Fromke, 1978).

ABORTION CAUSED BY COAGULATION DEFECTS

Recurrent abortion may occur due to congenital hypofibrinogenemia (Hahn *et al.*, 1978), lack of factor XIII (Egbring *et al.*, 1970) or in patients with lupus anticoagulant (Carreras *et al.*, 1981) along with impaired prostacyclin production. An intact fibrin network, diminished fibrinolysis and a physiological balance of thromboxane A_2 and prostacyclin could be important for placental implantation and vascularization.

HEMOSTATIC CHANGES WITH SEPTIC AND MISSED ABORTION

Septic abortion still has a high mortality rate of 0.4 to 0.6 deaths per 100 000 abortions (Grimes *et al.*, 1981). Coagulation changes with DIC – an early feature and complicating factor of endotoxin shock – are found in about 35 % of these patients (Grimes *et al.*, 1981).

Ascending intrauterine infection can cause release of endotoxins, platelet activation, acute disseminated intravascular coagulation and/or intensive intravascular hemolysis with consecutive septic shock and renal failure (Williams *et al.*, 1976). Hemolysis may be a result of fibrin deposition in the microvasculature (Bonnar, 1981; Kuhn and Graeff, 1979).

Coagulation profiles give positive soluble fibrin monomer complexes (SFMC) indicating increased thrombin activity (Table 10.1). Platelet activation is followed by thrombocytopenia. Fibrinogen is reduced. Activation of fibrinolysis causes elevated fibrin(ogen) degradation product (FDP) values (Pritchard and MacDonald, 1976; Kuhn and Graeff, 1979). Some authors suggest prophylaxis with low-dose heparin, which is considered to lower the risk of development of a DIC and hemorrhage (Kuhn and Graeff, 1979). A definite beneficial effect has not yet been generally accepted (Pritchard and MacDonald, 1976). Heparin given in therapeutic dosage to patients with depleted coagulation factors, aggravates any existing bleeding, especially if there are large wound areas like the placental insertion.

Table 10.1 Coagulation profiles in septic and missed abortion (SFMC = soluble fibrin monomer complexes, FDP = fibrin degradation products)

Component	Fibrinogen	Platelets	SFMC	FDP
Septic abortion	(↓)	↓ ↓	↑	↑
Missed abortion	↓	(↓)	↑	↑ ↑

(↓) = (slightly) decreased; (↑) = increased

Important therapeutic steps are immediate restoration and maintenance of the circulation, adequate antibiotics to control infection, and evacuation of the infected products of conception. Additional infusion of coagulation factors (fresh frozen plasma), is recommended, if necessary (Bonnar, 1981).

In cases of missed abortion, thromboplastic and fibrinolytic material from the dead products of conception are released into the materal circulation (Pritchard and MacDonald, 1976; Kuhn and Graeff, 1979). Coagulation and fibrinolysis are activated, resulting in a latent consumptive coagulopathy (Lerner *et al.*, 1967; Pfeifer, 1968). After 3–5 weeks the 'dead fetus syndrome' with consumptive coagulopathy is established in about 25 % of cases (Kuhn and Graeff, 1979). As long as no attempts to evacuate the uterus are undertaken, the impaired coagulation is clinically without symptoms, but blood may be found incoagulable when dilatation and evacuation or drug-induced abortion occurs. Coagulation changes in missed abortion are summarized in Table 10.1. Fibrinogen is usually low, platelet count tends to be reduced, SFMC are increased, plasminogen and antiplasmins decreased, and FDP are elevated (Bonnar, 1981; Briel *et al.*, 1978; Kuhn and Graeff, 1979; Pritchard and MacDonald, 1976). If consumptive coagulopathy is established, coagulation defects should be corrected by giving fresh frozen plasma prior to evacuation of the dead products of conception. The additional use of low-dose heparin and/or organic inhibitors of fibrinolysis such as aprotinin to block DIC and fibrinolysis may be considered (Bonnar, 1981; Kuhn and Graeff, 1979; Pfeifer, 1968; Pritchard and MacDonald, 1976).

COAGULATION CHANGES CAUSED BY DIFFERENT METHODS OF INDUCING ABORTION

Suction curettage for therapeutic abortion in the first trimester of pregnancy does not usually lead to changes in coagulation and fibrinolysis apart from a 40% decrease in factor XIII and a 50% decrease in platelet aggregation (Kidess *et al.*, 1979). These changes are found both with local and with general anesthesia.

Table 10.2 Hemostatic changes in abortion induced by suction curettage (first trimester), hypertonic solutions, oxytocin, Rivanol, PGE_2, $PGE_{2\alpha}$ and Sulprostone (second trimester)

	Coagulation	Fibrinolysis	Platelet aggregation
Suction curettage	nc (F XIII $\downarrow$)	nc	$\downarrow$
Hypertonic solutions	$\uparrow$ subclinical DIC	$\uparrow$	?
Oxytocin	($\uparrow$)	($\uparrow$)	($\uparrow$)
Rivanol	nc–($\uparrow$)	($\uparrow$)	?
PGE_2, $PGF_{2\alpha}$	nc–($\uparrow$)	($\uparrow$)	($F_{2\alpha}$) $\downarrow$
Sulprostone	nc	nc–($\uparrow$)	nc

nc = no change; ($\uparrow$) = (slightly) increased; ($\downarrow$) = (slightly) decreased

It is well established that intra-amniotic instillation of hypertonic solutions such as saline, urea, or glucose is regularly complicated by subclinical DIC (Burkmann *et al.*, 1977; MacKenzie *et al.*, 1975, Shaw and Ballard, 1974). The pathophysiology of DIC in these patients is still not clear. DIC may be caused by release of thromboplastic material from the uterus and its contents after administration of hypertonic solutions, which may cause cellular disruption in the products of conception (Talbert and Blatt, 1979).

A severe DIC with consumptive coagulopathy and hemolytic shock develops with a frequency of $1 : 400–1 : 1000$ (Talbert and Blatt, 1979). The additional use of oxytocin may increase the risk of significant DIC (Cohen and

Ballard, 1974). Coagulation profiles show typical changes consistent with DIC: factors I, V, VIII and platelets are low, and FDP high.

Oxytocin given intravenously, and in high dosage may be used alone or in combination with other drugs to induce missed abortion. It tends to activate both coagulation and the fibrinolytic system as well as platelet aggregation (Briel *et al.*, 1979). Rivanol given extra-aminiotically is not considered able to induce coagulation disorders (Ölund and Bistoleti, 1980).

Prostaglandins (PGE_2 and $PGF_{2\alpha}$) administered intra-amniotically, extra-amniotically or intravenously have little influence on coagulation, fibrinolysis and platelet function (Badraoui *et al.*, 1973; Briel *et al.*, 1978; Howie, 1976). Not only in therapeutic abortion, but also in patients with missed abortion in the initial stage of DIC, no signs of intravascular consumption of the coagulation system were found during or after the administration of $PGF_{2\alpha}$ (Briel *et al.*, 1978). Coagulation factors remain constant, or tend to increase. Fibrinolysis is activated to a small extent. There may be slight reduction in platelet aggregation due to oral PGE_2 (Myatt and Elder, 1975) and $PGF_{2\alpha}$ given intravenously (Briel *et al.*, 1978). Methyl-derivatives of $PGF_{2\alpha}$, administered intramuscularly have a similar effect on coagulation, fibrinolysis and platelet function as intravenous $PGF_{2\alpha}$ (Keirse *et al.*, 1980).

New synthetic prostaglandin derivatives, mostly PGE derivatives, with less marked systemic side effects and better efficacy due to a specific effect on the myometrium, have been introduced. Sulprostone, a PGE_2 derivative, can be given intravenously or intramuscularly. In therapeutic abortion and missed abortion, coagulation and fibrinolysis as well as platelet function remained constant (Briel and Lippert, 1981; Schander *et al.*, 1979).

CONCLUDING REMARKS

In therapeutic abortion hemostatic risks are small, and different methods for the evacuation of the uterus are advisable.

In septic abortion and missed abortion severe coagulation defects may develop. These should be corrected before evacuation of the uterus is undertaken, to avoid hemorrhage. The use of heparin and inhibitors of fibrinolysis must be considered cautiously. Intra-amniotic hypertonic solutions are not advisable as they may induce DIC. Thus, synthetic prostaglandin derivatives, which can be given systemically and have no adverse effects on hemostasis, are recommended.

References

Badraoui, M. H. H., Bonnar, J., Hillier, K. and Embrey, M. P. (1973). Blood coagulation changes during mid-trimester abortion induced by prostaglandin $F_{2\alpha}$. *Br. Med. J.*, **4**, 375–8

Bonnar, J. (1981). Haemostasis and coagulation disorders in pregnancy. In Bloom, A. L. and Thomas, D. P. (eds) *Haemostasis and Thrombosis*. pp. 454–71. (Edinburgh: Churchill Livingstone)

Briel, R. C. and Lippert, T. H. (1981). Biological action and half life in plasma of intramuscular sulprostone for termination of second trimester pregnancy. *Prostaglandins Med.*, **6**, 1–8

Briel, R. C., Kidess, E., Kunz, S. and Dieter, B. (1978a). Studies on platelet function during different modes of administration of PGF$_{2\alpha}$ in obstetrics and gynecology. *Arch. Gynäkol.*, **225**, 201–8

Briel, R. C., Kunz, S. and Kidess, E. (1978b). Influence on haemostasis excercised by prostaglandin F$_{2\alpha}$ in missed abortion. *Geburtsh. Frauenheild.* **38**, 862–7

Briel, R. C., Kunz., S. and Kidess, E. (1979). Platelet function, coagulation and fibrinolysis during termination of missed abortion and missed labor by PGF$_{2\alpha}$ and oxytocin. *Acta Obstet. Gynecol. Scand.*, **58**, 361–4

Burkmann, R. T., Bell, W. R., Atienza, M. F. and King, T. M. (1977). Coagulopathy with midtrimester induced abortion: Association with hyperosmolar urea administration. *Am. J. Obstet. Gynecol.*, **127**, 533–6

Carreras, L. D., Defreyn, G., Machin, S. J., Vermylen, J., Deman, R., Splitz, B. and van Assche, A. (1981). Arterial thrombosis, intrauterine death and "lupus" anticoagulant: detection of immunoglobulin interfering with prostacyclin formation. *Lancet*, **1**, 244–6

Cohen, E. and Ballard, C. A. (1974). Consumptive coagulopathy associated with intraamniotic saline instillation and the effect of intravenous oxytocin. *Obstet. Gynecol.*, **43**, 300–3

Egbring, R., Andrassy, K., Egli, H. and Mayer-Lindenberg, J. (1970). Untersuchungen bei zwei Patienten mit kongenitalem Faktor-XIII-Mangel. *Thromb. Diathes. Haemorrh.*, **23**, 313–39

Grimes, D. A. and Cates, W., Jr. (1979). Complications from legally-induced abortion: a review. *Obstet. Gynecol. Surv.*, **34**, 177–91

Grimes, D. A., Cates, W., Jr. and Selik, R. M. (1981). Fatal septic abortion in the United States, 1975–1977. *Obstet. Gynecol.*, **57**, 739–44

Guidotti, R. J., Grimes, D. A. and Cates, W., Jr. (1981). Fatal amniotic fluid embolism during legally induced abortion, United States, 1972 to 1978. *Am. J. Obstet. Gynecol.*, **141**, 257–61

Hahn, L., Lundberg, P. A. and Teger-Nilsson, A. C. (1978). Congenital hypofibrinogenaemia and recurrent abortion. *Br. J. Obstet. Gynaecol.*, **85**, 790–3

Harman, Ch. R., Fish, D. G. and Tyson, J. E. (1981). Factors influencing morbidity in termination of pregnancy. *Am. J. Obstet. Gynecol.*, **139**, 333–7

Howie, P. W. (1976). Prostaglandins and blood coagulation. In Karim, S. M. M. (ed.) *Prostaglandins: Physiological, Pharmacological and Pathological Aspects.* pp. 277–91. (Lancaster: MTP Press)

Keirse, M. J. N. C., Bennebroek-Gravenhorst, J., Boekhout-Mussert, M. J., Dubbeldam, J. and Veltkamp, J. J. (1980). Coagulation changes during management of fetal death with 15 (S)-15-methylprostagladin F$_{2\alpha}$. *Eur. J. Obstet. Gynecol. Reprod. Biol.*, **11**, 43–8

Kidess, E., Briel, R. C., Miller, H. and Dieter, B. (1979a). Das Verhalten der Thrombozyten-aggregation bei Schwangerschaftstermination während des ersten Trimesters. *Arch. Gynecol.*, **228**, 629–30

Kidess, E., Briel, R. C., Preissner, A. and Leipold, J. (1979b). Änderung der Faktor-XIII-Aktivität bei Schwangerschaftstermination mittels Saugkürettage. *Arch. Gynecol.*, **228**, 627

Koplik, L. (1977). Disseminated intravascular coagulation after a dilatation and evacuation abortion at 16 weeks' gestation. Annual Meeting, National Abortion Federation, Denver, Colorado

Kuhn, W. and Graeff, H. (eds.) (1979). *Coagulation Disorders in Obsterics.* (Stuttgart, New York: Thieme)

Lerner, R., Marqolin, M., Slate, W. G. and Rosenfeld, H. (1967). Heparin in the treatment of hypofibrinogenemia complicating fetal death in utero. *Am. J. Obstet. Gynecol.*, **97**, 373–8

MacKenzie, I. Z., Sayers, L., Bonnar, J. and Hillier, K. (1975). Coagulation changes during second-trimester abortion induced by intra-amniotic prostaglandin E$_2$ and hypertonic solutions. *Lancet*, **2**, 1066–9

Moberg, P., Sjöberg, B. and Wiqvist, N. (1975). The hazards of vacuum aspiration in late first trimster abortions. *Acta Obstet. Gynecol. Scand.*, **53**, 113–18

Myatt, L. and Elder, M. G. (1975). The effects on platelet aggregation of oral prostaglandin E$_2$ used for the induction of labour. *Br. J. Obstet. Gynaecol.*, **82**, 449–52

Ölund, A. R. and Bistoletti, P. (1980). Koagulations- und Fibrinolysesystem bei Rivanol-induziertem Schwangerschaftsabbruch. *Zbl. Gynäcol.*, **102**, 507–12

Pfeifer, G. W. (1968). Proteinasenblockade bei abgestorbener Schwangerschaft, "dead fetus syndrome". *Dtsch. Med. Wochenschr.*, **93**, 479–85

Pritchard, J. A. and MacDonald, P. C. (eds) (1976). *Williams Obstetrics.* pp. 426–8. (New York: Appleton-Century-Crofts)

Schander, K., Budde, U. and Bellmann, O. (1979). Untersuchungen zum Verhalten der plasmatischen Gerinnung und der Thrombozytenfunktion bei der Abortinduktion mit dem Prostaglandin E_2-Derivat Sulproston. *Arch. Gynecol.*, **228**, 635–7

Shaw, S. T., Jr. and Ballard, C. A. (1974). Subclinical coagulopathy following amnioinfusion with hypertonic saline. *Am. J. Obstet. Gynecol.*, **118**, 1081–8

Sromme, W. B. and Fromke, V. L. (1978). Amniotic fluid embolism and disseminated intravascular coagulation after evacuation of missed abortion. *Obstet. Gynecol.*, **52**, 1 (Suppl.), 76–80

Talbert, L. M. and Blatt, P. M. (1979). Disseminated intravascular coagulation in obstetrics. *Clin. Obstet. Gynaecol.*, **22**, 889–900

11
Complications of induced abortion

V. M. SADAUSKAS and V. J. CZIGREIENE

According to WHO data, some 50 million women in all countries seek induction of abortion (Husman, 1976; Stringer, 1974). Various methods for induction of abortion at different stages of pregnancy have been widely used in family planning (Czigreiene *et al.*, 1981; Grünberger and Riss, 1979; Havranek and Šmeral, 1979; Nemec *et al.*, 1978; Sadauskas and Czigreiene, 1979; Schott *et al.*, 1982; Schulze and Herold, 1978; Vaicekaviczene *et al.*, 1980; Vasiljev, 1979; Voigt *et al.*, 1977; Zwahr *et al.*, 1979). However, comparative studies of complications of early-induced abortions with those of late-induced abortions are rather scarce. The number of studies dealing with late complications of artificial abortions is smaller, despite the fact that their number increases with every year.

Late complications following artificial abortions include: endometrium damage, uterine cavity adhesions, uterotubal patency impairment, causing infertility, isoimmunization and psychogenic disorders occur in 10–35 % of the cases, and early ones in 5–20 % (Bräuutigam and Koller, 1979; Hale *et al.*, 1979; Kirchoff, 1977; Mandelin and Karjalainen, 1979; Nemec *et al.*, 1978; Schulze and Herold, 1978).

Our aim was to investigate the incidence and character of complications of induced abortions according to the duration of pregnancy, and the method of abortion induction used at the same center.

The normal structure of the cervix and isthmus of the uterus is important for the physiological course of pregnancy. Changes in their structure lead to spontaneous abortion due to the incompetence of the uterine internal orifice (Czigreiene *et al.*, 1981; Grünberger and Riss, 1979; Kirchoff, 1977; Mandelin and Karjalainen, 1979; Schott *et al.*, 1982; Voigt *et al.*, 1977). Patients who have had operations involving mechanic dilatation of the cervical canal and uterus curettage, may later develop impairment of the uterus-closing apparatus leading to its incompetence, premature delivery of subsequent pregnancy or habitual abortion (Obel, 1979; Zwahr *et al.*, 1979).

The rate of low-mass newborns weighing less than 2500 g amounts to 10.7 % among women who previously had pregnancy termination, as opposed to a 5 % rate among those who had no pregnancy termination (Zwahr *et al.*, 1979). This index increases to 9.5 % for women who indicate only pregnancy cessation in anamnesis, 12 % for those who had only premature labor, and

24 % for women with history of premature labor and interrupted pregnancy. Induced abortions are increasing each year (Tyler, 1981).

Special techniques for termination of pregnancy were being elaborated so as to diminish the possibility of damaging the cervix uteri (Atienza et al., 1975; Edelman et al., 1974; Sadauskas and Czigreiene, 1979; Stringer, 1974; Vaicekaviczene et al., 1980; Vasiljev, 1977, 1978). Presently, one method used involves a vacuum aspiration in early pregnancy without resorting to cervix dilatation (Edelman et al., 1974; Sadauskas, 1979, 1980; Stringer, 1974; Van de Vlugt et al., 1976; Vasiljev, 1977, 1978). This method decreases the rate of complications (1–3.8 %), because the cervical canal is not traumatized by forced dilatation (Edelman et al., 1974; Grünberger and Riss, 1979; Stringer, 1974; Vasiljev, 1977; Voigt and Seewald, 1975). Inflammatory complications are met only in 1–2 % (Sadauskas and Czigreiene, 1979; Vasiljev, 1977, 1978); cervical shock in 7 %. In 86–90 % of the cases, bleeding may occur after this procedure (Janaud et al., 1979; Vasiljev, 1977, 1978) and subsequent menstruation occurs after 4–5 weeks.

According to the WHO data, the rate of premature labors (WHO Scientific Group Report) and spontaneous abortions in cases of vacuum aspiration is much lower than in those cases where metal dilators are used.

The outcome of induced abortions is analyzed in 6586 women, divided into two groups according to the method used for induction of abortion. Group 1 consisted of 5220 women who had vacuum aspiration without cervix dilatation in outpatient conditions during the period of menses disappearance for no more than 14 days. A plastic cannula (Fig. 11.1) from 4.5 to 6 mm in diameter was used for this purposes. Before the procedure the cervical canal is smeared with 2 % Sol. Dicaini or 2–5 % Sol. Trimecaini. The cervix is fixed with atraumatic forceps. The cannula is passed up to the fundus uteri and then

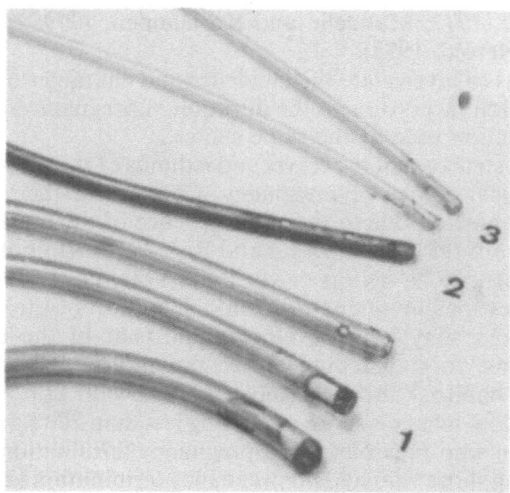

Fig. 11.1 Plastic cannulas

moved forward and backward, turning along the axis to 180°. At the same time the cannula acts as a uterine probe. At its end there are openings on opposite sides for suction of the uterine substance. The cannula is pulled out when one is sure that vacuum aspiration is finished; i.e. when there is a sensation of a "crunch of snow" and the bubbles in the system are noticed.

Group 2 consisted of 1366 women who underwent cervix dilatation by means of metallic dilators. Vacuum aspiration was then performed, the gestational age being from 6 to 12 weeks. Overnight hospitalization is required. The patient is intravenously anesthetized with Sombrevin or thiopental-Na.

Women from 21 to 30 years of age showed the highest rate of pregnancy termination.

In the first group nulliparous women made up 8.6 %, while in the second group they made up 7.8 % of the cases.

Table 11.1 shows that unmarried women, who terminated pregnancy, in the first group made up 8.6 % of the cases, and in the second group they made up 7.8 % of the cases. Therapeutic abortion in Group 1 was performed in 1.7 % of the cases and in Group 2 in 12 % of the cases. Complications of vacuum aspiration in Group 1 were not observed, while in Group 2 there were 2 cases of perforation of the isthmic part of the uterus caused by dilatation using Hegar's dilators. The uterus was sutured and the patients left the hospital in good health. All complications in both groups were divided into three types: early complications (during the first 7 days after pregnancy termination); late complications (from day 8 until 30 days); and the so-called 'latent' complications observed during subsequent pregnancy, labor and the post-natal period.

The total number of complications in Group 1 was observed in 88 cases (1.7 %) (Table 11.2), and in Group 2 in 71 cases (5 %) (Table 11.3).

Tables 11.2 and 11.3 show that early complications in Group 1 were observed in 1.1 % of the cases and in Group 2 in 2.7 % of the cases. Among early complications, inflammation occurred in 0.2 % of the cases in Group 1

Table 11.1 Reasons for interruption of pregnancy

	Group 1		Group 2	
The reason	No. of cases	Percentage	No. of cases	Percentage
1. Single	451	8.6	107	7.8
2. Having one child	2001	38.3	126	9.2
3. With two children	2158	41.3	358	26.2
4. With three children	187	3.6	89	6.5
5. With four children	135	2.6	18	1.3
6. Lives away from husband	92	1.8	29	2.1
7. Single having a baby	90	1.7	190	14.0
8. Feeling unwell	5	0.1	34	2.5
9. Extragenital pathology	87	1.7	165	12.1
10. Other reasons	14	0.3	250	18.3
Total:	5220	100.0	1366	100.0

Table 11.2 Complications after vacuum aspiration, Group 1

Complications	No. of cases		Percentage		
Early complications					
Repeated aspiration	48 ⎫		0.9 ⎫		⎫
Acute endometritis	4 ⎬ 59		0.1 ⎬ 0.2		⎬ 1.1
Exacerbation of chronic salpingitis	7 ⎭		0.1 ⎭		⎭
Late complications					
Ectopic pregnancy	4 ⎫		0.1 ⎫		
prolonged bleeding	15 ⎬ 29		0.3 ⎬		0.6
Unsuccessful pregnancy termination	10 ⎭		0.2 ⎭		
Total	88				1.7

Table 11.3 Complications after induced abortion, Group 2

Complications	No. of cases		Percentage		
Early complications					
Acute endometritis	13 ⎤		1.0 ⎱ 1.9		⎤
Exacerbation of chronic salpingitis	12		0.9 ⎰		
Intensive bleeding during the procedure	6 ⎬ 36		0.4		⎬ 2.7
Uterine perforation	2		0.2		
Sensitivity to Sombrevine	3 ⎦		0.2		⎦
Late complications					
Chorion residue	15 ⎤		1.0		⎤
Hematometra	10		0.7		
Subinvolution of uterus	4 ⎬ 35		0.3		⎬ 2.5
Thrombophlebitis at the site of injection	4		0.3		
Salpingitis tumorosa	2 ⎦		0.2		⎦
Total	71				5.2

and in 1.9 % of the cases in Group 2. Late complications in the first group were observed in 0.6 % of the cases, and in the second group in 2.6 % of the cases. Delayed bleeding was the most frequent late complication occurring in the first group (in 0.3 % of the cases). Chorion residue occurred in 1.0 % of the cases in Group 2 and hematometra in 0.7 % of the cases.

Analyzing 'latent' complications, infertility was observed in 0.1 % of the cases in Group 1, and in 3 % of the cases in Group 2.

Pregnancy and labor was analyzed in 160 women in Group 1 and in 120 women in Group 2.

After vacuum aspiration – performed before day 14 – discharge of secretions are observed on the 3rd–4th day, which usually is not observed when pregnancy is interrupted beyond 12 weeks using cervix dilatation. This may be due to the fact that during vacuum aspiration not all mucosa is evaluated, and it is discharged from the uterus within 3–4 days. Subsequent normal mesntruation takes place after 4–5 weeks. Bleeding during vacuum aspiration is not abundant: in Group 1 it averaged 27.7 ±11 ml, lasting for 4 ±3.5 min, and in Group 2 100.7 ±ml, lasting for 7.8 ±12 min.

Basal temperature taken during 536 menstruation cycles showed that in Group 1 it was biphasic in 93.7 % of the cases, monophasic in 6 %, and of 305 cycles in Group 2 it was biphasic in 76 % of the cases and monophasic in 23.7 % of cases.

In Group 1 the character of the first menstruation cycle following pregnancy termination showed no changes in 37.5 % of cases, and in 62.5 % of cases menstruation cycles changed: in 90.0 % they became longer than usual, but not abundant. Subsequent cycles were still unchanged. In Group 2 changes of menstruation cycle were observed in 57.2 %.

For establishing cervical incompetence, isthmography was done for 42 women in Group 1 and for 50 women in Group 2.

Roentgenograms of women in Group 1 showed that the cervical canal was thin, with its length equal to the length of the uterus, and the width of the canal was not more than 2–3 mm. (Fig. 11.2a).

Roentgenograms of women in Group 2 (Fig. 11.2b) showed that in 42 cases the length of the cervical canal was decreased in comparison with the length of the uterine cavity, and increased in the width of the cervical canal of the uterus by more than 6 mm, particularly in the isthmic part of the uterus.

Pregnancy termination by vacuum aspiration without dilatation of the cervical canal before day 14, is less traumatic and has more advantages over pregnancy termination using mechanical dilatation of the cervical canal of the uterus. Studies in this field are in progress.

It is important to note some aspects in the psychological status of patients. In Group 1 about 80 % of women were afraid of the pain that may be involved, when subjected to it for the first time, and only 15 % of the women were afraid of the repeated procedure. Almost 90 % of the women felt fine after this procedure, and only 10 % felt pain in the lower part of the abdomen, which disappeared in 2–3 h.

In conclusion, pregnancy termination by means of vacuum aspiration has more advantages over the widely spread method using mechanical means for dilatation and curettage. Such advantages may be: slight bleeding, rapidity of the procedure, absence of cervix and uterus traumatization, simplicity of the technique, absence of anesthetic risk, absence of uterus perforation risk, slight

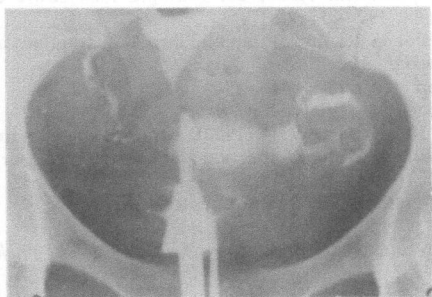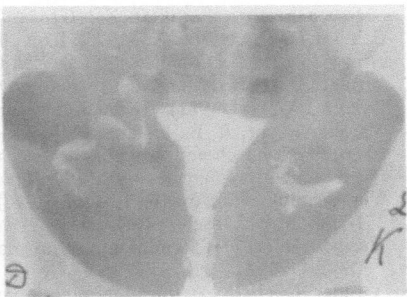

Fig. 11.2 (a) Roentgenogram: the uterus canal after vacuum aspiration without damage. (b) Roentgenogram: changes in the uterus canal when Hegar's dilators were used

impairment of the hormonal balance, minimal complications and preservation of the capacity for work. Vacuum aspiration used in the early stages of gestation can be viewed as a means of prevention of premature labor.

References

Atienza, M. F., Burkman, R. T., Burnett, L. S. *et al.* (1975). Menstrual extraction. *Am. J. Obstet. Gynecol.*, **121**, 490–5

Bräuutigam, H. H. and Koller, S. (1979). Statistische Erhebungen über Komplikationen nach Schwangerschftsabbruch in der Bundesrepublik Deutschland. *Arch. Gynecol.*, **228**, 344–8

Bräuutigam, H. H. and Warnke, W. (1981). Zur Häufigkeit von Spätkomplikationen des legalen Schwangerschaftsabbruches in der Bundesrepublik Deutschland. *Z. Geburtsh. Perinatol.*, **185**, 193–9

Czigreiene, V. J., Vaicekaviczene, A. B. and Vilimene, P. M. (1981). Investigation of uterine cervical canal following artificial termination of pregnancy. Abstracts Congress of Obst. Gynecol. of Lithuanian SSR. Vilnius, pp. 95–6

Edelman, D. A., Brenner, W. E. and Goldsmith, A. (1974). Menstrual Regulation (MR) in four countries. Introduction. *IPPF Med. Bull.*, **8**, 1–2

Grünberger, W. and Riss, P. (1979). Isthmozervikale Insuffiziennz nach vorangegangener Zerwixdilatation und Kürettage. *Wien Med. Wochenschr.*, **129**, 390–2

Hale, R. W., Kobara, T. Y., Sharma, S. D. *et al.* (1979). Office Termination of pregnancy by "menstrual aspiration". *Am. J. Obstet. Gynecol.*, **134**, 213–18

Havranek, F. and Šmeral, P. (1979). Prerušeni ranych stadii tehotenstivi (regulace menstruace miniinterruyce)v praxi. *Čs. Gynecol.*, **44**, 561–6

Husman, C. (1976). Menstrual regulation: patient selection and the results of series. *New Developments in Fertility Regulation.* pp. 28–32 (Virginia: Airline House)

Janaud, A., Relia, D. *et al.* (1979). Regulation menstruelle. *Gynecologie*, **30**, 239–43

Kirchoff, H. (1977). Schwangerschaftsabbruch und Perinatal Medizin. *Geburtsch. Frauenheilkd.*, **37**, 849–56

Mandelin, M. and Karjalainen, O. (1979). Pregnancy outcome after previous induced abortion. *Ann. Chir. Gynecol.*, **68**, 147–54

Nemec, D. K., Prendergast, T. J. and Trumbowez, W. D. (1978). Medical abortion complications: an epidemiologic study at a mid-Missouri clinic. *Obstet. Gynecol.*, **51**, 433–6

Obel, E. B. (1979). Pregnancy complications following legally induced abortion. *Acta Obstet. Gynecol. Scand.*, **58**, 485–90

Sadauskas, V. M. and Czigreiene, V. J. (1979). Vacuum aspiration of uterine mucosa in outpatient clinic. Actual problems of physiology and pathology of female generative function. *Charkov*, 67–8

Schott, G., Ehrig, E. and Wulff, H. (1982). Prospektive Untersuchungen der nachfolgenden Schwangerschaft nach induziertem und spontanem Abort bei Primigraviden sowie die Beurteilung der Fertilität. *Zbl. Gynäkol.*, **104**, 397–404

Schulze, G. and Herold, C. (1978). Komplikationen der Interruptio und ihre Auswirkungen auf nachfolgende Schwangerschaften. *Zbl. Gynäkd.*, **100**, 1261–5

Stringer, J. (1974). Menstrual regulation. Conference in Hawaii. *IPPF Med. Bull.*, **8**, 3.

Tyler, C. W., Jr. (1981). Epidemiology of abortion. *J. Reprod. Med.*, **26**, 459–69

Vaicekaviczene, A. B., Sadauskas, V. M. and Czigreiene, V. J. (1980). Atraumatic pregnancy termination techniques as a method decreasing incidence of abortion and premature labour in subsequent pregnancies. *Premature Labour*, (Moscow), p. 85

Van de Vlugt, Piotrow, P. T. *et al.* (1976). Menstrual regulation update. *Pop. Report*, ser. F. No. 4, May, Wasch., pp. 49–64

Vasiljev, D. (1977). Termination of pregnancy at early terms modo N. Karman. *Akuš.i ginekol* (Sofia), 74–81

Vasiljev, D. (1978). Artificial termination of pregnancy at early terms modo N. Karman. *Akuš.i ginekol* (Sofia), **17**, 98–103.

Voigt, R. and Seewald, H. J. (1975). Zur Frage des Kausalzusammenhangs zwischenn Interruptio und nachfolgenger vorzeitiger Schwangerschaftsbeendigung. *Zbl. Gynäkol.*, **97**, 1375–7

Voigt, R., Seewald, H. J. and Voigt, P. (1977). Klinische Untersuchungen zum Kausalzusammenhand zwischenn Abruptio und nachfolgender Geburt eines untergewichtigen Kindes. *Z. Geburtsh. Perinat.*, **181**, 438–47

Weathersbee, P. S. (1980). Early reproductive loss and the factors that may influence its occurrence. *J. Reprod. Med.*, **25**, 315–18

World Health Organization Scientific Group Report (1979). World Health Organization Technical Report Series No. 623

Zwahr, Ch., Voigt, M., *et al.* (1979). Mehrdiemensionale Untersuchungen zur Prüfung von Zusammenhängen zwischenn Interruptioanamnese und Frühgeburtenanamnese und der Geburt von "Kinder mit niedrigem Geburtsgewicht". *Zbl. Gynäkol.*, **101**, 1502–9

12
Effects of spontaneous and induced abortions on subsequent pregnancies and fetal outcome

N.KLEARCHOU, J. BONTIS and S. MANTALENAKIS

The effect of spontaneous and induced abortions on subsequent pregnancy and labor is not well documented. Evidence exists for a clear correlation between abortions and premature labors though this issue is strongly debated (Hogue, 1974; Kotasek, 1975; Funderburk et al., 1975; Voigt et al., 1976).

Since induced abortion still exists in Greece as the main method of family planning, the study of the problem is of great importance. The purpose of this study was to present and evaluate our data on this issue.

During a 3-year period (1977–79) 685 premature labors were registered in a total of 4885 women who entered our clinic for labor. The parameters used for premature newborns were the gestational age (26–36 weeks) and the newborn's weight (800–2500 g). In all women studied we looked for first or second trimester abortions – spontaneous or induced – and the correlation found with premature labors was statistically analyzed, using Student's t-test.

Of the 4885 women included in the study, 1683 admitted spontaneous or induced abortions (Table 12.1). In-term newborns were delivered by 1297 of these 1683 women (77 %) and by 2903 of the 3202 without abortion (91 %) (Table 12.1). The difference found (14 %) was of high significance ($p = 0.01$). When the mother's age was taken in account this difference was still significant, though it admittedly was lower in the subgroup of women aged less than 20 ($p = 0.04$) (Table 12.2). When parity was analyzed as an

Table 12.1 The incidence of premature and in-term newborns in correlation with spontaneous and induced abortions

	No. of cases	Premature new borns		In-term newborns	
		n	Percentage	n	Percentage
Spontaneous abortions	645	164	26	481	75
Induced abortions	1038	222	21	816	79
No abortions	3202	299	9	2903	91

Table 12.2 The effect of mother's age on the percentage of the in-term labors in correlation with previous spontaneous and induced abortions

	Mother's age (in years)		
	< 20	21–30	> 30
	In-term newborns (%)		
Spontaneous abortions	82*	· 72**	75***
Induced abortions	80*	76**	82***
No abortions	90*	89**	95***

* $p = 0.04$; ** $p = 0.01$; *** $p = 0.01$

additional factor the results showed a significant difference to exist between the 2-para. and 3-para. concerning spontaneous abortions and between primipara and all multipara concerning induced abortions (Table 12.3).

The onset of labor – namely contractions, premature rupture of membranes (PRM) and bleeding – was also correlated with previous abortions both in the group of premature and at-term labors. In both groups abortions have been shown to have an inverse correlation with contractions and a positive one with PRM, and the differences were of statistical significance (Tables 12.4 and 12.5). Further analysis showed a strong positive correlation to exist between PRM and induced rather than spontaneous abortions, particularly in the group of premature labors (Table 12.5). In-term labors risk for PRM was definitely lower even when an abortion – induced or spontaneous – was present in the gynecological history of the woman (Table 12.4). Results were also of statistical significance. When total incidences of PRM and contractions were mutually compared in the group of prematures a large increase was noticed in women who had admitted abortion

Table 12.3 The incidence of in-term labors in primipara and multipara in relation to previous abortions

No. of labors		No. of cases	No. of in-term newborns	Percentage
1	Spontaneous abortion	197	146	74
1	Induced abortion	240	160	66
1	No abortion	1518	1366	90
2	Spontaneous abortion	231	190	82
2	Induced abortion	379	306	80
2	No abortion	1288	1175	91
3	Spontaneous abortion	140	93	66
3	Induced abortion	270	230	85
3	No abortion	299	264	88
4	Spontaneous abortion	77	52	67
4	Induced abortion	149	120	80
4	No abortion	110	102	92

Table 12.4 The incidence of contractions, premature rupture of membranes (PRM) and bleeding in at-term labors in relation to previous abortions

	Contractions		PRM		Bleeding	
	n	Percentage	n	Percentage	n	Percentage
Spontaneous abortion	415	59	183	39	6	0.14
Induced abortion	359	51	148	32	5	0.12
All abortions	774	54	466	35	11	0.26
No abortions	1857	64	638	22	6	0.14
Total	2569	62	1105	26	17	0.40

Table 12.5 The incidence of contractions, premature rupture of membranes (PRM) and bleeding in premature labors in relation to previous abortions

	Contractions		PRM		Bleeding	
	n	Percentage	n	Percentage	n	Percentage
Spontaneous abortion	55	34	76	46	33	20
Induced abortion	65	29	118	53	44	20
All abortions	120	31	194	50	77	20
No abortions	120	40	34	65	65	21
Total	240	35	296	43	142	21

(Table 12.5), suggesting that a possible cervical incompetence, probably due to previous abortion, led to premature labor, at least in this group of pregnant women.

Another remarkable point is that in this same group of premature newborns the incidence of bleeding seems not to be dependent on previous abortions, though it is significantly higher in premature rather than in-term labors taken as a whole (Tables 12.4 and 12.5). If abortion's causal relation to premature labor is to be accepted, the above data could be interpreted as evidence that abortion acts as a factor leading indirectly to bleeding.

Premature labor is of diverse etiology. Bleeding, pre-eclampsia, twin pregnancy, uterus malformations and rhesus incompatibility are regarded as being among the commonest etiological factors. Furthermore, parameters such as age, social class, number of previous labors, parent's body size, embryo's sex and mother's smoking during pregnancy seem to be of critical importance for gestational duration.

Induced abortions, though illegal and condemned by religion, are still the main method of family planning in Greece. Their effect of subsequent pregnancy remains a point of controversy. A two-fold increase in premature labors in women with past abortions has been found by two different groups in Greece (Pantelakis et al., 1973; Papaevangelou et al., 1973). Furthermore a ten-fold increase of second trimester miscarriages in pregnancies which followed an induced abortion has been described, and frequent clinical evaluation has been proposed as a mean for early diagnosis of cervical incompetence (Wright et al., 1972).

This correlation, however, could not be proved in other studies (Daling, 1975; Roht and Aoyama, 1974; Van der Slikke and de Treffers, 1978) and instead of abortion other parameters, such as social class, number of previous pregnancies, mother's age and a history of past intrauterine deaths have been proposed as responsible for premature labors (Daling, 1975). In our study a positive correlation between gestational age and abortions – induced or spontaneous – did exist regardless of mother's age, though women whose age ranged from 21 to 30, and those older than 30, were shown to be more vulnerable compared to women under 20, in whom, however, the correlation was still significant ($p = 0.04$).

A significant decrease of in-term labors in 3-para. and 4-para. with previous spontaneous abortions was found in our cases, though a worse effect on multipara has been described by other authors (Gardiner *et al.*, 1978). On the other hand, concerning induced abortions an increased incidence of premature labors has been shown by our findings in primipara compared to multipara, and the difference found was significant. These data could be interpreted as evidence that the adverse effects of induced abortions are most deleterious on the first pregnancy rather than on subsequent ones. Significant differences concerning the onset of labor have also been found in our study. The increased incidence of PRM in prematures was probably due to cervical incompetence. Thus a positive correlation between abortions – whether induced or spontaneous – and premature labors seems to be valid. Furthermore, abortions are related to an increased incidence of PRM in the group of prematures, while in women with no abortions this correlation does not exist. Cervical incompetence seems not to be the cause of premature labor in the later case, where contraction frequency is higher. The degree of cervix dilatation and the different techniques used for an abortion may be critical factors for subsequent pregnancies. Vacuum curettage, leading to minimal cervix dilatation, seems to carry a better prognosis. Abortion seems to be not only an out-of-date method of family planning, but also a dangerous one.

Data from 4885 consecutive labors were analyzed to determine the effect of previous spontaneous and induced abortion on premature rupture of membranes (PRM) and prematurity. The study was made over a 3-year period. Women with premature labor were compared with other women of similar gravity or parity who terminated their pregnancy. The incidence of prematurity was extremely higher in women with one or more abortions – induced or spontaneous – when it was compared to women without abortions. The incidence of PRM was significantly higher in premature labors. Cervical incompetence is though to be the cause of premature labor in the group of women with abortions.

References

Daling, J. R. (1975). Induced abortion and subsequent outcome of pregnancy. *Lancet*, **26**, 170–2

Funderburk, S. J., Guthrie, D. and Meldrum, D. (1975). Suboptimal pregnancy outcome among women with prior abortions and premature births. *Am. J. Obstet. Gynecol.*, **126**, 55–60

Gardiner, A., Clarke, C., Cowen, J., Finn, R. and McKendrick, O. M. (1978). Spontaneous abortion and fetal abnormality in subsequent pregnancy. *Br. Med. J.*, **1**, 1016–18

Hogue, C. J. (1974). Low birth weight subsequent to induced abortion. A historical prospective study of 948 women in Skopje, Yugoslavia. *Am. J. Obstet. Gynecol.*, **123**, 675–81

Kotasek, A. (1975). In Stembera, Z. K. *et al.* (eds.) *4th European Congress of Perinatal Medicine, 1974.* p. 183. (Stuttgart: Thieme)

Pantelakis, S. N., Papadimitriou, S. G. and Doxiadis, S. A. (1973). Influence of induced and spontaneous abortions on the outcome of subsequent pregnancies. *Am. J. Obstet. Gynecol.*, **116**, 799–805

Papaevangelou, G., Vrettos, S. A., Papadatos, C. and Alexiou, D. (1973). The effect of spontaneous and induced abortion on prematurity and birthweight. *J. Obstet. Gynaecol. Br. Commonw.*, **80**, 418–22

Roht, L. H. and Aoyama, H. (1974). Induced abortion and its sequelae: prematurity and spontaneous abortion. *Am. J. Obstet. Gynecol.*, **120**, 868–74

Van der Slikke, I. W. and De Treffers, P. E. (1978). Influence of induced abortion on gestational duration in subsequent pregnancies. *Br. Med. J.*, **1**, 270–2

Voigt, R., Seewald, H. J. and Starker, K. (1976). Klinische und röntgenologische Untersuchungen zur Frage des Zusammenhangs zwischen Interruptio und Frühgeburt. *Zbl. Gynäkol.*, **98**, 1589–93

Wright, C. S. W., Campbell, S. and Beazléy, J. (1972). Second-trimester abortion after vaginal termination of pregnancy. *Lancet*, **10**, 1278–9

13

Prophylactic antibiotics in induced abortion

L. HEISTERBERG, S. SONNE-HOLM and J. T. ANDERSEN

The majority of voluntary interruptions of pregnancy (VIP) are performed on young, healthy women. Many are concerned with the risk of acute complications as well as possible sequelae. Their physicians should be able to give adequate information, not only in the form of general rates, but with numbers pertaining to each individual woman based on her age, parity, social and economic status, the current technique of abortion and the gestational age of her pregnancy. Since many sequelae are caused by post-abortal genital infection it is important to know the frequency of this acute complication, its significance, and to delineate possible risk groups which may benefit from antibiotic prophylaxis.

In 1976 VIP was performed at a rate of 22 per 1000 women between 15 and 44 years of age in the USA, and from 18 to 26 per 1000 in the Scandinavian countries. The highest rates of VIP were reported from Cuba, 71; Bulgaria, 66; and Hungary, 42. The lowest rate for Europe was noted in Scotland, i.e. 8. The total number of abortions in 1976 exceeded 1 million in the USA alone (WHO, 1978).

INFECTIOUS MORBIDITY AFTER VOLUNTARY INTERRUPTION OF PREGNANCY

Frequencies

The frequencies of infectious morbidity after VIP varied in the literature, and comparisons are difficult because of differences in populations, techniques, definitions of genital infections, types of follow-up , and gestational ages. Often, population characteristics such as age and parity are not stated in the reports, nor are complications related to age groups, social classes, etc. The rate of certain complications varies according to the abortion technique employed. The range of gestational ages also differs from area to area, and this clearly influences the complication rate, as it is associated with gestational age.

Reports from the last decade comprising population characteristics, techniques applied, definitions of complications, and gestational age groups,

Table 13.1 Frequencies of infectious morbidity following legal abortion, including the 12th gestational week, in studies with and without follow-up with a pelvic examination

No. of patients	Definition of infection	Rate of infection (%) Without follow-up	With follow-up	Reference
4733	+	0.7		Andolsek, 1974
3411	+	3.3		Burkman et al., 1976
810	−	1.4		Harman et al., 1981
10453	−	0.2		Hodgson and Portmann, 1974
26000	+	1.5		Nathanson, 1972
53880	−	1.4		Tietze and Lewit, 1972
110	+	15.5		Weström et al., 1981
1228	−		1.6[1]	Jerve and Fylling, 1978
106	+		10.4	Krohn, 1981
291	+		12.8[2]	Meirik et al., 1981
1123	+		7.2	Moberg et al., 1975
239	+		10.9	Sonne-Holm et al., 1981
270	+		11.9	Westergaard et al., 1982

[1] 90% of patients had follow-up
[2] 83% of patients had follow up

including the 12th week, gave frequencies of infectious morbidity after VIP of 0.2–15.5% when there was no follow-up with a pelvic examination. (Table 13.1). When follow-up with pelvic examinations was performed, the frequencies ranged from 1.6 to 12.8% (Table 13.1). Follow-up data are of Scandinavian origin and are based on a rather small number of patients. The fact that a woman does not return to the physician who performed the abortion does not mean the post-operative course was uncomplicated. Consequently, the frequencies given in the studies without follow-ups must be evaluated as minimal figures.

The possible role of subclinical infections following VIP is unknown, but may be elucidated by paired serological tests demonstrating a rise in specific antibodies, e.g. to *C. trachomatis*, *M. hominis*, etc. (Mårdh, 1980).

Mortality

Mortality rates per 100 000 legal abortions vary from country to country, partly due to differences in the stage of gestation at which abortions are performed. The rate in the USA for 1975 was 2.6, and was 2.7 in Denmark for the period 1967–76 (WHO, 1978). Abortion mortality increases continuously with advanced gestational age, being 0.6 per 100 000 abortions at 8 weeks or less gestational age, 4.9 at 11–12 weeks, and 25.2 at 16 weeks for all methods employed in the USA during the years 1972–75. Infection was the main cause of 28 out of a total of 104 deaths associated with legal abortions in America for that period (Grimes and Cates, 1979).

Ectopic pregnancies

Post-abortal genital infections such as pelvic inflammatory disease (PID) have been associated with an increased risk of subsequent ectopic pregnancies. The

114

problem is poorly investigated. Two case–control studies comparing the frequencies of previous VIP in women treated for ectopic pregnancy and in controls have given contradictory information. One study (Andolsek, 1974) reported that the risk of ectopic pregnancy was the same in women with a history of legal abortion as in controls. Another study (Panayotou et al., 1972) observed a significantly higher frequency of ectopic pregnancy in women with positive histories of induced, illegal abortions. In two retrospective studies the frequency of ectopic pregnancy in women who have and have not had a previous VIP has been compared, giving conflicting results; i.e. a significant difference versus no difference (Koller and Eikhorn, 1977; Dalaker et al., 1979).

Studies of this nature are unable to relate post-abortal genital infections to a possible increased danger of subsequent ectopic pregnancy.

Fertility

Information is contradictory on possible sterility after legal abortion. No significant difference in fertility after legal abortion has been found (Roht and Aoyama, 1974; Hogue, 1975). Women with post-abortal PID have a significantly longer period with failure to conceive than women without this complication (Obel, 1979). As the study only included women who have become pregnant following VIP, the frequency of infertility could not be estimated, and only suggested that PID following a legally induced abortion may lead to decreased fertility. After illegally induced abortion a relative risk of infertility has been found (Trichopoulos et al., 1976).

Valid prospective investigations without bias in patient selection and comparison of women with and without post-abortal PID are needed to give an idea of the frequency of infertility subsequent to post-abortal infection.

Other sequelae

PID can give rise to pelvic pain, either in the form of chronic pelvic pain, dyspareunia, or dysmenorrhea. The possible association between induced abortion complicated with PID and pelvic pain has never been mentioned when sequelae to VIP were discussed.

RISK FACTORS

Microbial flora

To justify the administration of prophylactic antibiotics, identification of groups which carry a significant risk of post-surgical infection is mandatory. Until recently induced abortion has been considered a procedure with so low an incidence of infectious morbidity that prophylaxis was thought to be clinically irrelevant. Lately, however, groups of women have been found to carry a risk of post-abortal infection at a rate justifying antibiotic prophylaxis.

Women with untreated endocervical gonorrhea have a significantly increased danger for post-abortal endometritis (Burkman *et al.*, 1976). Gonococcal culture results should be obtained before abortion. Women harboring *C. trachomatis* in their cervix at the time of abortion have a significantly increased frequency of post-abortal PID compared with women in whom this organism was not found (Møller *et al.*, 1982; Qvigstad *et al.*, 1982; Westergaard *et al.*, 1982). The frequencies ranged from 20 to 28 %. All studies recommended that women should be cultured for *C. trachomatis* before abortion, and antibiotics administered to those with positive cultures.

Cervical cultures yield a vast spectrum of the microbial flora, most of which are not responsible for post-abortal PID. It is difficult to single out the responsible organisms. The problem has been clearly demonstrated in several studies (Andolsek, 1974; Krohn, 1981; Moberg *et al.*, 1978) where no association between the pre-abortal cervical microbial flora and post-abortal infection could be found. Moberg *et al.* concluded that cultivation of the cervical microbial flora cannot predict which patients will develop subsequent genital infection.

History of pelvic inflammatory disease

In a prospective trial (Sonne-Holm *et al.*, 1981) women with previous PID run a significantly increased risk (22 %) of contracting post-abortal infection. A history of gonorrhea was significantly more frequent among *Chlamydia*-positive than among *Chlamydia*-negative women (Westergaard *et al.*, 1982). The groups of women with a history of PID and with *Chlamydia*-positive cervical cultures may overlap to a large extent. Institutions unable to perform *Chlamydia* cultures should be able to identify many of these women by their history. Inquiring about a previous PID is a simple, rapid, and cheap way of detecting a patient at risk.

Gestational age

There is uncertain evidence regarding the role of gestational age upon the rate of infectious morbidity after abortion. Many authors find an increased frequency of complications with advanced gestational age but do not distinguish between complications such as hemorrhage, perforation of the uterus, retained placental tissue, and pelvic infection. The highest incidence of pelvic infection has been found at or earlier than the 8th week of gestation among 1228 abortions, but no statistical tests were employed (Jerve and Fylling, 1978). The gestational age influenced the rate of infection, the frequency being significantly higher in the 11–12-week gestational-age group compared with the 6–7- and 8–10-week gestational-age groups. The effect of prophylaxis was not correlated with this variable (Sonne-Holm *et al.*, 1981).

In contrast, other studies (Moberg *et al.*, 1975; Tietze and Lewit, 1971) found no clearcut correlation of post-abortal infection with gestational age, although the latter reported incidences of pelvic infections in local patients of 0.9 % for a gestational age of up to 8 weeks, 1.2 % for 9–12 weeks, and 1.6 % for gestational ages 13 weeks and above.

Other risk factors

Few studies specifically relate rates of post-abortal infection with age, parity, abortion method, type of anesthesia, application of an IUD, or socioeconomic status.

In one study (Jerve and Fylling, 1978) the highest incidence of pelvic infection was found among women below 20 years of age and in nulliparous women. The differences were small and no significance tests were employed.

Dilatation and curettage compared with the suction method entail no differences in infection rates after VIP (Andolsek, 1974; Jurukovski and Sukarov, 1971). Frequencies of genital infection varied between 0.7 and 1.7%, the total number of patients in the two studies being 23 000.

The use of different types of cannulas in vacuum aspiration has been evaluated in two studies (Antonovski *et al.*, 1975; Andolsek *et al.*, 1976). Three types of cannula, metal versus flexible plastic (Karman) and flexible plastic (Karman) versus non-flexible plastic, gave frequencies of pelvic infection of 2.7 versus 8.0% (significantly different) and 8.0 versus 6.9% (not significantly different). The only other significant difference with regard to complication was a higher rate of retained tissue obtained with the flexible plastic than with the non-flexible plastic cannula.

Infection rates after VIP, using local or general anesthesia, seem controversial. One controlled trial (Andolsek *et al.*, 1977) observed PID frequencies of around 2% with non-significant differences. A large prospective study (Grimes *et al.*, 1979), comprising a total of 54 000 women who received local or general anesthesia for suction curettage, demonstrated local anesthesia to be associated with higher rates of febrile morbidity, although both anesthetic techniques had similar aggregated major complication rates.

Immediate post-abortal intrauterine device insertion is not associated with any increased danger of genital infection (Goldsmith *et al.*, 1972; Newton *et al.*, 1974; Burkman *et al.*, 1977; Sonne-Holm *et al.*, 1981).

Heisterberg *et al.* (1982) found no correlation between age, parity, number of previous spontaneous and induced abortions, social status, and the occurrence of post-abortal PID.

SELECTIVE PROPHYLAXIS

Non-randomized reports on prophylactic antibiotics (Table 13.2)

Although the seven reports presented in Table 13.2 comprise a total of 100 000 legal abortions, it is difficult to establish a clear picture of the frequency of post-abortal genital infection and the effect of prophylactic antibiotics. The frequency among non-treated women varied between 0.07 and 20% and was not listed in one report. Two of the works only gave rates for the total material, and statistical tests were employed in only three. Control groups were used in just four of the studies, in which one administered placebo treatment. There were large differences in methods with regard to patient follow-up and administration of prophylaxis. Two of the studies included follow-ups. Most authors administered systemic antibiotics with tetracycline

Table 13.2 Non-randomized reports on the prophylactic use of antibiotics on women undergoing legal abortion

Method	No. of patients	Antibiotics	Rate of infection (untreated treated; %)	Reference
On all	62 620	Not stated	0.3[1]	Beric et al., 1973
On all	10 890	Tetracycline	Not stated	Bozorgi, 1977
On women with previous PID and unmarried				Jurukovski and Sukarov, 1971
< 25 years	18 758	Sulfonamide	1.3[1]	
Controlled	4000	Tetracycline	9/3	Hodgson et al., 1975
Controlled, placebo	2950	Doxycycline	0.07/0.6	Brewer, 1980
On women with Chlamydia, controlled	943	Doxycycline	22/0	Møller et al., 1982
Controlled	490	Vaginal chloro-quinaldol	13/9	Meirik et al., 1981

[1] Rate for total number of patients

or derivatives, but for periods varying from 1 to 4 days. In one study the antibiotic prescribed was not stated, while one report assessed vaginal prophylaxis. Three studies employed methods which permitted valid conclusions to be drawn with regard to the effect of prophylaxis. One (Brewer, 1980) found a significant reduction of post-abortal infection with doxycycline, and another (Møller et al., 1982) demonstrated a significant reduction of infection in women harboring C. trachomatis when given doxycycline. The third study (Meirik et al., 1981) detected no significant effect of vaginal chloroquinaldol on post-abortal infection.

Randomized studies on prophylactic antibiotics (Table 13.3)

In a double-blind trial (Krohn, 1981) the effect of a single, pre-operative oral dose of 2 g tinidazole was assessed. Of 106 women randomized to the placebo group, 10.4 % developed a pelvic infection, and of 104 in the tinidazole group 5.8 % developed infection. Tinidazole given pre-operatively seems to reduce the incidence of pelvic infection after abortion. No statistical analysis

Table 13.3 Randomized double-blind studies on the prophylactic use of antibiotics on women undergoing legal abortion

Reference	No. of patients	Antibiotics	Rate of infection (placebo/active; %)
Krohn, 1981	210	Trinidazole	10/6
Weström et al., 1981	212	Trinidazole	16/10
Sonne-Holm et al., 1981	493	Penicillin G + pivampicillin	11/6 (22/2)[1]

[1] Numbers in parentheses pertain to rate of infection for women with a history of PID.

accompanied the results, but by application of the χ^2 test the difference was found to be non-significant ($p > 0.20$).

In another Swedish study with similar design and antibiotic regimen (Weström et al., 1981), incidences of pelvic infection were 15.5% in the placebo group and 9.8% in the treatment group, a non-significant difference.

A study comprising 493 women, of whom 254 were randomized to treatment with 2 million IU of penicillin intramuscularly $\frac{1}{2}$ h before, and again 3 h after, abortion followed by 350 mg pivampicillin t.d.s. for 4 days and 239 for placebo treatment, found post-abortal pelvic infection incidence to be 5.5% in the antibiotic group and 10.9% in the placebo group. This difference could be attributed to the effect among women with a history of PID, of whom 22.4% contracted pelvic infection compared with 7.2% among women without previous PID. The effect of prophylactic antibiotics could be demonstrated only in the group with previous PID, in which the incidence was reduced to 2.1% ($p = 0.006$). The use of antibiotic prophylaxis could be considered justified in this group of women.

Selection of patients (Table 13.4)

Most of the frequencies of infectious morbidity after VIP reported in the literature seem to be of a magnitude which does not justify general prophylaxis. This concept is to a certain degree supported by the findings in most of the randomized or controlled trials, where antibiotic prophylaxis does not significantly reduce the frequency of post-abortal infections in the population as a whole. Some trials, however, seem to have disclosed groups of women with increased danger of contracting post-abortal PID that can be identified pre-operatively (Burkman et al., 1976; Møller et al., 1982; Qvigstad et al., 1982; Sonne-Holm et al., 1981; Westergaard et al., 1982). These groups comprise women with positive cervical cultures for gonococci, women with positive urethral and/or cervical cultures for C. trachomatis, and women with a history of PID. The effect of antibiotic prophylaxis has been demonstrated in the two latter groups of patients (Møller et al., 1982; Sonne-Holm et al., 1981). With regard to women with gonorrhea gonococci should be cultured before abortion and the women treated when necessary.

Surgical procedures involving contaminated surfaces are often associated with transient bacteremia, e.g. women undergoing suction abortion (Ritvo et al., 1977; Heisterberg et al., 1983). Consequently, the Committee on Prevention of Rheumatic Fever and Bacterial Endocarditis of The American Heart Association has considered the problem in relation to patients with underlying heart disease (Kaplan et al., 1977). Dilatation and curettage of the uterus does not require antibiotic prophylaxis. Since a patient with a prosthetic valve appears to be at especially high risk, the Committee found that it may be wise to administer antibiotic prophylaxis with this procedure.

This statement is in accordance with the findings in our study (Heisterberg et al., 1983), where the administration of penicillin G 2 million IU intramuscularly $\frac{1}{2}$ h before abortion did not prevent bacteremia. However, prophylactic antibiotics may still prevent bacterial endocarditis, but demon-

Table 13.4 Recommendations for the use of antibiotic prophylaxis on women undergoing legal abortion

On women having	Drug	Dosage	Start/duration	Reference
Positive culture for N. gonorrheae	Procaine penicillin G[1] + probenicid	4.8 mill IU intramuscularly 1 g orally	Before abortion/ single dose	WHO, 1981
Positive culture for C. trachomatis	Doxycycline	100 mg/day	Before abortion/ 14 days	Møller et al., 1982
History of PID after abortion	Penicillin G + pivampicillin	2 mill IU 350 mg t.d.s. orally	$\frac{1}{2}$ h before and 3 h after abortion / Following penicillin/ 4 days	Sonne-Holm et al., 1981
Prosthetic heart valve	Penicillin G[2] + gentamycin	2 mill IU intramuscularly 1.5 mg/kg intramuscularly	Before abortion/ single dose / Before abortion/three doses every 8 hours	Kaplan et al., 1977

[1] Patients who are allergic to penicillin should be treated with oral tetracycline or spectinomycin 2 g intramuscularly
[2] Patients who are allergic to penicillin are given vancomycin 1 g intravenously over 30–60 min plus streptomycin 1 g intramuscularly. The dose of these antibiotics may be repeated in 12 h

stration of clinical effect on a rare event such as bacterial endocarditis will be very difficult and ethically questionable.

Adverse effects

The risks of possible adverse effects following use of all medicines must also be considered when antibiotics are administered prophylactically. For example, allergic reactions to penicillin can be fatal and prophylactic administration according to a standing instruction makes it even more imperative to check for any allergic inclination in all patients. Moreover, patients should be informed as to which drug they have received, and warned of possible side effects – preferably in writing.

The prescription of antibiotics on a wider scale always raises the question of the development of superinfection with resistant micro-organisms and the development of general resistance to the drug applied. The risk seems to be very small, but to meet such an emergency with effective antibiotics the prophylaxis should preferably be a single drug in common usage. With regard to the development of general resistance, one must bear in mind that the administration of any antibiotic prophylaxis should not only prevent clinical infection and thus reduce duration of hospitalization and costs; it should also lower the total amount of antibiotics poured into the microbial environment and thus keep the development of bacterial resistance at a minimum (Hirschmann and Inui, 1980). Unfortunately, only few studies involving antibiotic prophylaxis have focused attention on the possible change of resistance patterns of micro-organisms during a period with administration of a certain antibiotic, or estimated and compared the amounts of antibiotics administered with and without prophylaxis. None of the studies mentioned here has performed such a calculation. One study (Grossman *et al.*, 1977) tabulated the patterns of antibiotic resistance of *E. coli* isolates to cephalothins on the gynecological service, and those of the remainder of other services in the hospital, in an attempt to determine the effect of a clinical trial with antibiotic prophylaxis in pelvic surgery on the gynecological resident flora. The increase in *E. coli* cephalothin resistance on the gynecological service did not appear to be greater than the increase throughout the remainder of the hospital. It is recommended that institutions considering antibiotic prophylaxis should conduct epidemiological surveillance of resident flora and patterns of infection to ensure that prophylaxis is beneficial to its recipients without being detrimental to others. Another study on prophylaxis in Cesarean section (Gall, 1979) recorded total antibiotic use and found that the prophylactic group required less post-operative antimicrobial therapy for infectious complications. Because the prophylaxis was a four-dose course, the total amount of antibiotic administered was greater than in the placebo recipients.

Future studies on antibiotic prophylaxis in abortion should report the amount of antimicrobial agents used in treated and placebo groups, in order to permit an assessment of whether the nosocomial flora is receiving more or less ecologic pressure from the use of prophylaxis than would occur by the otherwise unprevented pelvic infections.

CONCLUDING REMARKS

With regard to timing of prophylactic antibiotics it has been demonstrated (Burke, 1961) that there is a definite period, beginning the moment the bacteria gain access to the tissue and lasting 3 h, during which infection may be suppressed by antibiotics. Thus prophylactic antibiotics produce maximum suppression of infection if they are present in the tissue when the microorganisms arrive. Depending on the route of administration and the drug, the prophylaxis in elective abortion should commence at a time which allows the drug to reach at least minimal inhibitory concentration for the known pathogens in the pelvic organs. However, it is not too late to start the prophylaxis during the procedure if one encounters unsuspected contamination.

The duration of prophylaxis has been debated. One review (Chodak and Plaut, 1977) stated that systemic prophylaxis longer than 2–3 days post-operatively cannot be justified. It is not known whether there is any value to extending prophylaxis beyond the first day or two (Shapiro et al., 1979). Hirschmann and Inui (1980) reported that adequate tissue levels of the antimicrobial agent probably need to be maintained only for the duration of the operation, and that post-operative prophylaxis actually represents early treatment.

Only two or three of the studies on prophylaxis in abortion (Tables 13.2 and 13.3) had limited antibiotic administration to pre-operative dosage. This could have been due to the fact that the endometrium through the cervical canal is in connection with the vagina and its flora, and is thus potentially contaminated for a longer period than a sutured wound. Further studies are needed to evaluate short-term versus long-term prophylaxis in induced abortion.

The total dose of a drug depends on duration and dosage. Single doses, however, need not normally be larger than necessary to ensure sufficient concentration in the target organs. If only a single dose is given pre-operatively, a larger dose than usual may be contemplated, depending on the half-life of the drug. Thus, two of the randomized trials on prophylaxis in abortion gave 2 g of tinidazole before abortion (Krohn, 1981; Weström et al., 1981). Such a dose will maintain therapeutic levels for approximately 24 h (Templeton, 1976). This is really a masked way of extending the duration of prophylaxis.

When selecting one or several drugs for prophylaxis, the ideal method is to find a chemotherapeutic agent which will kill all the bacteria responsible for the infection. Several investigators (Burkman et al., 1977; Andolsek, 1974; Moberg et al., 1978; Weström et al., 1981; Krohn, 1981; Heisterberg et al., 1983) have performed cervical cultures from women before abortion, as well as from women presenting with post-abortal endometritis. It is questionable whether such cervical cultures represent the flora responsible for the post-abortal endometritis, parametritis, and/or salpingitis. Most of these cases are caused by infectious agents ascending from the cervix, and can spread from iatrogenic complications, such as legal abortion (Mårdh, 1980). Microbiological findings in PID obtained by sampling from the uterus, cul-de-sac, or tubes most often comprise organisms such as *N. gonorrheae, C.*

trachomatis, M. hominis, U. urealyticum, and anaerobes. Percentages of recovery vary, depending on differences in sampling techniques, sites, and microbiological methods, but geographic differences may also play a role. These factors must be taken into consideration when deciding on a chemotherapeutic agent. In geographical areas where *C. trachomatis* is prevalent, such as Scandinavia, the tetracyclines or derivatives seem appropriate, as they too are effective against *M. hominis, U. urealyticum,* and *N. gonorrheae.* However, the prevalence of tetracycline-resistant *N. gonorrheae* and *U. urealyticum* may vary from area to area. Erythromycin has no effect on *M. hominis,* but is active against *N. gonorrheae, U. urealyticum* and *C. trachomatis* and most Gram-negative anaerobes (*Bacteroides* species), although increased levels of resistance have been demonstraed *in vitro* for a few strains of *C. trachomatis* (WHO, 1981). In areas with prevalent anaerobes, agents such as nitroimidazole derivatives, klindamycin, and lincomycin may be of value. Whether these drugs can act alone in prophylaxis remains to be proven. It is generally recommended to combine these drugs with other chemotherapeutic agents.

The third generation of cephalosporins, such as cephamandol and cefoxitin, have extended the spectra of action especially against anaerobes, both Gram-positive (*Chlostridia* species) and Gram-negative. They still have the same spectrum and the low toxicity of the penicillins.

The aminoglycosides are effective on Gram-negative rods and *Staph. aureus,* but not on anaerobes and most diplococci.

It is certainly of importance that future studies on prophylaxis in abortion test the effectiveness of different antibiotics with regard to immediate pelvic infections and also to long-term sequelae.

References

Andolsek, L. (ed.) (1974). *The Ljubljana Abortion Study.* (Ljubljana)

Andolsek, L., Miller, E. and Bernard, R. (1976). A comparison of flexible and nonflexible plastic cannulae for performing first trimester abortion. *Int. J. Gynaecol. Obstet.,* **14,** 199–204

Andolsek, L., Cheng, M., Hren, M., Ogrinc-Oven, M., Ng, A., Ratnam, S., Belsey, M., Edström, K., Heiner, P., Kinnear, K. and Tietze, C. (1977). The safety of local anesthesia and outpatient treatment: a controlled study of induced abortion by vacuum aspiration. *Fam. Plann. Perspect.,* **8,** 118–124

Antonovski, L., Ljatkova, K., Sukarov, L. L., Brenner, W. E., Edelman, D. A. and Bernard, R. P. (1975). A comparative study of metal and plastic (Karman) cannulae for first trimester abortion by suction curettage. *Int. J. Gynaecol. Obstet.,* **13,** 33–8

Beric, B., Kupresanin, M. and Kapor-Stanulovic, N. (1973). Accidents and sequelae of medical abortions. *Am. J. Obstet. Gynecol.,* **116,** 813–21

Bozorgi, N. (1977). Statistical analysis of first-trimester pregnancy terminations in an ambulatory surgical center. *Am. J. Obstet. Gynecol.,* **127,** 763–8

Brewer, C. (1980). Prevention of infection after abortion with a supervised single dose of oral doxycycline. *Br. Med. J.,* **281,** 780–1

Burke, J. F. (1961). The effective period of preventive antibiotic action in experimental incisions and dermal lesions. *Surgery,* **50,** 161–8

Burkman, R. T., Tonascia, J. A., Atienza, M. F. and King, T. M. (1976). Untreated endocervical gonorrhea and endometritis following elective abortion. *Am. J. Obstet. Gynecol.,* **126,** 648–51

Burkman, R. T., Tonascia, J. A., Atienza, M. F. and King, T. M. (1977). The relationship of immediate post-abortal intrauterine device insertion to subsequent endometritis: a case–control study. *Conception,* **15,** 435–44

Chodak, G. W. and Plaut, M. E. (1977). Use of systemic antibiotics for prophylaxis in surgery. A critical review. *Arch. Surg.*, **112**, 326–34

Dalaker, K., Lichtenberg, S. M. and Okland, G. (1979). Delayed reproductive complications after induced abortion. *Acta Obstet. Gynecol. Scand.*, **58**, 491–4

Gall, S. A. (1979). The efficacy of prophylactic antibiotics in cesarean section. *Am. J. Obstet. Gynecol.*, **134**, 506–11

Goldsmith, A., Goldberg, R., Eyzaguirre, H., Lucero, S. and Lizana, L. (1972). IUD insertion in the immediate postabortal period. In Goldsmith, A. (ed.) *Excerpta Med.* Family Planning Research Conference (Amsterdam)

Grimes, D. A. and Cates, W., Jr. (1979). Complications from legally-induced abortion: a review. *Obstet. Gynecol. Survey*, **34**, 177–91

Grimes, D. A., Schulz, K. F., Cates, W., Jr. and Tyler, C. W., Jr. (1979). Local versus general anesthesia: which is safer for performing suction curettage abortion? *Am. J. Obstet. Gynecol.*, **135**, 1030–5

Grossman, J. H., Adams, R. L. and Hierholzer, W. J. (1977). Epidemiologic surveillance during a clinical trial of antibiotic prophylaxis in pelvic surgery. *Am. J. Obstet. Gynecol.*, **128**, 690–2

Harman, Ch. R., Fish, D. G. and Tyson, J. E. (1981). Factors influencing morbidity in termination of pregnancy. *Am. J. Obstet. Gynecol.*, **139**, 333–7

Heisterberg, L., Sonne-Holm, S., Andersen, J. T., Hebjørn, S., Dyring-Andersen, K. and Hejl, B. L. (1982). Risk factors in first-trimester abortion. *Acta Obstet. Gynecol. Scand.*, **61**, 357–60

Heisterberg, L., Sonne-Holm, S., Sebbesen, O., Andersen, J. T., Hebjørn, S. and Dyring-Andersen, K. (1983). Prophylactic antibiotics and bacteremia in induced first-trimester abortions: a controlled trial. (Submitted)

Hirschmann, J. V. and Inui, T. S. (1980). Antimicrobial prophylaxis: A critique of recent trials. *Rev. Infect. Dis.*, **2**, 1

Hodgson, J. E. and Portmann, K. C. (1974). Complications of 10,453 consecutive first-trimester abortions: a prospective study. *Am. J. Obstet. Gynecol.*, **120**, 802–7

Hodgson, J. E., Major, B., Portmann, K. C. and Quattlebaum, F. W. (1975). Prophylactic use of tetracycline for first trimester abortions. *Obstet. Gynecol.*, **45**, 574–8

Hogue, C. J. (1975). Low birth weight subsequent to induced abortion. *Am. J. Obstet. Gynecol.*, **123**, 675–81

Jerve, F. and Fylling, P. (1978). Therapeutic abortion. *Acta Obstet. Gynecol. Scand.*, **57**, 237–40

Jurukovski, J. and Sukarov, L. L. (1971). A critical review of legal abortion. *Int. J. Gynaecol. Obstet.*, **9**, 111–17

Kaplan, E. L., Anthony, B. F., Bisno, A., Durack, D., Houser, H., Millard, H. D., Sanford, J., Shulman, S. T., Stillerman, M., Taranta, A. and Wengler, N. (1977). Prevention of bacterial endocarditis. *Circulation*, **56**, 139A–143A

Koller, O. and Eikhorn, S. N. (1979). Late sequelae of induced abortion in primigravidae. *Acta Obstet. Gynecol. Scand.*, **56**, 311–17

Krohn, K. (1981). Investigation of the prophylactic effect of tinidazole on the postoperative infection rate of patients under-going vacuum aspiration. *Scand. J. Infect. Dis.*, Suppl. 26, pp. 101–3

Mardh, P.-A. (1980). An overview of infectious agents of salpingitis, their biology, and recent advances in methods of detection. *Am. J. Obstet. Gynecol.*, **138**, 933–51

Meirik, O., Nilsson, S. and Nygren, K.-G. (1981). Vaginal application of a chemotherapeutic agent before legal abortion. *Acta Obstet. Gynecol. Scand.*, **60**, 233–5

Moberg, P., Sjöberg, B. and Wiqvist, N. (1975). The hazards of vacuum aspiration in late first trimester abortions. *Acta Obstet. Gynecol. Scand.*, **54**, 113–18

Moberg, P., Eneroth, P., Harling, J., Ljung, Å and Nord, C.-E. (1978). Preoperative cervical microbial flora and postabortion infection. *Acta Obstet. Gynecol. Scand.*, **57**, 415–19

Møller, B. R., Ahrons, S., Laurin, J. and Mårdh, P.-A. (1982). Pelvic infection after abortion associated with *Chlamydia trachomatis*. *Obstet. Gynecol.*, **59**, 210–13

Nathanson, B. N. (1972). Ambulatory abortion: experience with 26,000 cases (July 1, 1970, to August 1, 1971). *N. Engl. J. Med.*, **286**, 403–7

Newton, J., Elias, J. and Johnson, A. (1974). Immediate post-termination insertion of copper 7 and Dalkon shield intrauterine contraceptive devices. *J. Obstet. Gynaecol. Br. Commonw.*, **81**, 389–92

Obel, E. B. (1979). Fertility followng legally induced abortion. *Acta Obstet. Gynecol. Scand.*, **58**, 539–42

Panayotou, P. P., Kaskarelis, D. B., Miettinen, O. S., Trichopoulos, D. B. and Kalandidi, A. K. (1972). Induced abortion and ectopic pregnancy. *Am. J. Obstet. Gynecol.*, **114**, 507–10

Qvigstad, E., Skaug, K., Jerve, F., Ulstrup, J. C. and Fylling, P. (1982). Therapeutic abortion and *Chlamydia* infection. *Contraceptive Delivery Systems*, **3**, 531

Ritvo, R., Monroe, P. and Andriole, V. T. (1977). Transient bacteremia due to suction abortion: implications for SBE antibiotic prophylaxis. *Yale J. Biol. Med.*, **50**, 471–9

Roht, L. H. and Aoyama, H. (1974). Induced abortion and its sequelae: prematurity and spontaneous abortion. *Am. J. Obstet. Gynecol.*, **120**, 868–74

Shapiro, M., Townsend, T. R., Rosner, B. and Kass, E. H. (1979). Use of antimicrobial drugs in general hospitals. Patterns of prophylaxis. *N. Engl. J. Med.*, **301**, 351–5

Sonne-Holm, S., Heisterberg, L., Hebjørn, S., Dyring-Andersen, K., Andersen, J. T. and Hejl, B. L. (1981). Prophylactic antibiotics in first-trimester abortions: a clinical controlled trial. *Am. J. Obstet. Gynecol.*, **139**, 693–6

Templeton, R. (1976). Metabolism and pharmacokinetics of metronidazole: a review. In Finegold, S. M. (ed.) *Proceedings of the International Metronidazole Conference.* (Amsterdam: Excerpta Medica)

Tietze, C. and Lewit, S. (1971). Legal abortion: early medical complications. *Fam. Plann. Perspect.*, **3**, 6–14

Tietze, C. and Lewit, S. (1972). Joint program for the study of abortion (JPSA): early medical complications of legal abortion. *Fam. Plann. Perspect.*, **3**, 97–122

Trichopoulos, D. B., Handanos, N., Danezis, J., Kalandidi, A. K. and Kalaputhaki, V. (1976). Induced abortion and secondary fertility. *Br. J. Obstet. Gynaecol.*, **83**, 645–50

Westergaard, L., Philipsen, T. and Scheibel, J. (1982). Significance of cervical Chlamydia trachomatis infection in postabortal pelvic inflammatory disease. *Obstet. Gynecol.*, **60**, 322–5

Weström, L., Svensson, L., Wölner-Hanssen, P. and Mårdh, P.-A. (1981). A clinical double-blind study on the effect of prophylactically administered single dose tinidazole on the occurrence of endometritis after first trimester legal abortion. *Scand. J. Infect. Dis.*, Suppl. 26, pp. 104–9

World Health Organization (1978). Induced abortion. Technical Report Series 623. (Geneva)

World Health Organization (1981) Nongonococcal urethritis and other selected sexually transmitted diseases of public health importance. Technical Report Series 660. (Geneva)

Part IV

Psychosocial Aspects

14
Legal aspects of scientific research on fetuses in The Netherlands

E. M. DERKS-HAMMELBURG, W. A. A. VAN OS and P. E. R. RHEMREV

DUTCH LAW

Dutch law finds its origin in Roman law, and is applicable in most of Europe. The following information may not be entirely applicable in countries with laws of Anglo-Saxon origin.

HUMAN RIGHTS

Human rights begin at birth and end at death. Although physicians can manipulate the actual moment of birth and death, these essential events in human existence have legal significance.

The law distinguishes between biological and legal life (1.3). Biological life exists before birth and may persist after death. Such life is not entitled to personal rights. This does not mean that legal rights are not given to life before birth or to the body after death. Prior to birth the fetus is protected, and after death the human body remains the object of rights. This protection differs from that of human beings from the time of their birth to their death.

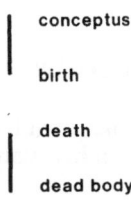

conceptus

birth

death

dead body

BIRTH

Under Dutch law, birth is defined as the moment a person's name is recorded on a birth certificate. A birth certificate is issued exclusively for live-born infants. Under civil law, being born alive is the decisive factor. The fetus is granted rights only as necessary (*nasciturus pro iam nato habetur*). Only then can it be the holder of subjective rights. For example, it can become heir to the father who died during the pregnancy.

THE FETUS

The fetus in the womb is not a legally recognized human being; however, this does not mean that all legal protection is withheld from it. At what moment is it possible to speak in legal terms of a fetus?

Under Dutch law, legal protection of the fetus starts at nidation. At that time it is considered a 'pregnancy' or 'a fetus with which the woman is pregnant'. Even though in the legal sense the fetus is not a human being, it does have legal significance. In civil as well as in criminal law, there are rules with regard to the fetus carried by a woman. For example: in case the husband of a pregnant woman dies, a curator is to be appointed to the unborn fetus (*curator ventris*).

The fetus has a separate legal status from the mother. Together they form an entity, but the fetus is not a part of the mother's body. The mother can die with the fetus surviving, and vice-versa.

ABORTED FETUS

Should the live fetus produced by *abortus procatus* be regarded as having been born? The law is not very clear with regard to live-born fetuses. Of course, at the time these laws were enacted, current abortion practices were not taken into consideration. A fetus produced by abortion may be regarded as: aborted (penal code), born (civil code) or not born if it is less than 24 weeks old (Law on the Disposal of Dead Bodies).

A term frequently used in this connection is 'viable', i.e. capable of independent life. A fetus capable of independent life must be kept alive. Whether a fetus is capable of independent life is decided by the physician who performs the abortion.

PROTECTION AFTER ABORTION

A woman's right with regard to her own body does not include the fetus, and extends only to its presence within her womb. The mother cannot subject the fetus to medical experiments.

When a woman decides to have a legal abortion she no longer places her body at the disposal of the fetus. She has that right under certain circumstances. The pivotal question with regard to abortion is not whether the woman has the right to kill the fetus, but whether she has the right to terminate her care of the growing fetus. Therefore, where abortion is concerned one should not speak of the right to kill. The consequence of this is that if an independently viable fetus is aborted, it may not be killed. Legally, this fetus has been born and the woman is not entitled to demand the death of the fetus.

Scientific research

Scientific research in medicine is justified to broaden existing knowledge which may eliminate, alleviate or prevent disease and suffering. It is only permitted when it meets legal requirements.

LAW AND SCIENTIFIC RESEARCH

Intervening with dead or live bodies involves rights of the person, or of those entitled to dispose of the dead body. As a result, explantation and autopsy cannot be performed unless the legal requirements are fulfilled with regard to the rights of the live donor, the deceased person, or his next of kin. A person's body is his property. This gives him full rights over that body; rights which do not terminate upon death. The question whether, after death, the body becomes the property of the heirs has not been settled by Dutch law. The closest relatives must give their permission to open the body and remove any organs from it, unless the subject decided differently before he died.

Autopsy

Autopsy, obduction, post-mortem examination and partial dissection are opening of a body and possible removal of the parts for diagnosis or verification of a diagnosis. Autopsy is regulated in the Law on the Disposal of Dead Bodies. Permission must be granted by the subject (codicil) or his next of kin.

This system differs from that of other countries, such as France, where the criterion is the no-objection system, i.e. permission is assumed unless expressly denied.

Extirpation

Extirpation (explanation, transplantation) is the removal of organs, tissues or substances from a body on behalf of someone else, or for research purposes. Organs may be extirpated from a live donor (hair, blood, sperm) or from a dead body (kidneys, cornea).

When does a body die? Under Dutch law the criterion for death is the cessation of brain function. The removal of organs is permissible when such cessation occurs, regardless of the possibility of the continuing function of the heart and the respiratory organs. It is even permissible for purposes of explanation to keep a dead body functioning by artificial means. Questions of transplantation have not been settled officially by Dutch law. The same rules are used that apply to autopsies.

Experiments

An experiment is an observation to increase scientific knowledge through new methods. The legality of such experiments depends on two criteria: reasonableness and granted permission.

In order to fulfill the criterion of reasonableness the experiment must provide new insights and betterment of science of the community. The experiment must be in accordance with scientific principles and be based on adequate research. It must be performed by scientifically qualified persons; the subject's mental and physical suffering must be limited, etc. Many of the conditions imposed on the performance of experiments have been included in the 'Helsinki Declaration'.

Scientific research on aborted fetuses

Increased knowledge of human growth and development prior to birth has produced a desire to carry out research involving embryos and fetuses. The importance of such research is that it affords insight into prenatal development of organs, into genetic problems and into fetal physiology, which will promote the elaboration of prophylactic techniques to help endangered fetuses during pregnancy and parturition, etc.

Dead fetus

A dead fetus is a still-born fetus. If the still-born fetus is immature, it is regarded under Dutch law as not having been born. It may be placed at the disposal of the physician by derelictio (i.e. the gaining of proprietorship by abandonment) under the proprietorship by abandonment law. The physician has the right to dissect the fetus and to remove organs, tissue or substance from it.

In the case of a still-born, but mature, fetus, burial is obligatory. To perform autopsy or extirpate organs it is necessary to obtain permission from the mother as the closest relative present at the time of death.

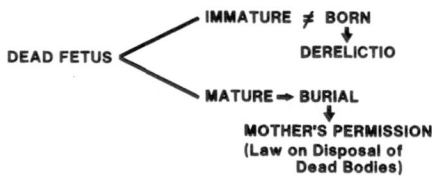

LIVE-BORN, NOT INDEPENDENTLY VIABLE FETUS

This fetus has its own legal status, which does not depend on whether or not it has been aborted. The woman does not have the right to dispose of the fetus, just as parents do not have the right to dispose of their children.

The Dutch Supreme Court ruled in 1960 that the Law on the Disposal of Dead Bodies also applies to immature fetuses which lived after birth and subsequently died. The mother's permission is required for autopsy and extirpation after the death of such fetuses.

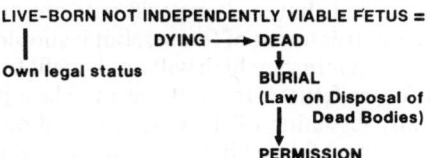

```
LIVE-BORN NOT INDEPENDENTLY VIABLE FETUS =
        |             DYING ───► DEAD
        |                        |
  Own legal status              BURIAL
                                (Law on Disposal of
                                |      Dead Bodies)
                                |
                                PERMISSION
```

LIVE-BORN, INDEPENDENTLY VIABLE FETUS

A live-born fetus acquires the rights of a person. Experiments on such fetuses are only permissible for therapeutic reasons after obtaining permission from the parents. In all other cases such experiments constitute a punishable offense (assault or possibly manslaughter or murder). If the child dies at a later date, heirs other than the mother may also grant permission for autopsy and extirpation.

```
           LIVE-BORN INDEPENDENTLY VIABLE FETUS
                      |
           BORN ─► CERTIFICATE ─► DEAD ─► BURIAL
             |                      |
       SUBJECT OF LAW         MOTHER'S PERMISSION
                 |
          HEIRS' PERMISSION
```

INTRAUTERINE FETUS

The rule that neither the mother nor both parents can give permission for experimentation on live-born fetuses applies also to the intrauterine fetus. Interventions involving fetuses which have a therapeutic purpose are not experiments. Administration of antibiotics to protect the fetus from syphilis is an example. An experimental element may be introduced here by treating two fetuses with two different antibiotics in order to determine which has the better placental passage. Provided both antibiotics are capable of bringing about the desired effect, such an experiment need not be unlawful. The criterion is that the activity involved will be harmless.

Because such an experiment is being conducted in the mother's body, it is necessary for the mother to be informed in detail and to give her consent (informed consent).

Since the legal status of the fetus in the womb is not affected by the question of whether or not abortion has been decided upon, it is irrelevant to distinguish between experiments *in utero* on fetuses which will be delivered normally and fetuses which will be aborted. Experiments of this nature should, therefore, preferably not be carried out in an abortion clinic. If the experimental group includes women who desire an abortion, the abortion must not be postponed for reasons concerned with the experiment; nor must the abortion procedure be altered.

Even during these harmless experiments, the greatest caution should be exercised.

It is frequently asserted that such experiments are necessary for scientific progress in the prenatal treatment of fetuses; but it should be kept in mind that research is being done on fetuses which will not benefit from it, since the object is the treatment of future fetuses. In itself this may be a justifiable motive, but it does not justify any lessening of the care which should be exercised while conducting experiments on fetuses in the womb, even if these experiments are harmless.

Those concerned should realize that they are liable in the case of adverse affects!

CONCLUDING REMARKS

Most abortions involve still-born, immature products of conception. There are no problems with scientific research on, and extirpation of, organs from these products of conception, under Dutch law. In all other cases, mature still-born fetuses, live-born fetuses mature or immature and viable or non-viable, fetuses, permission must be obtained from the mother or heirs before an autopsy can be performed or explanting organs, substances or tissues can be done.

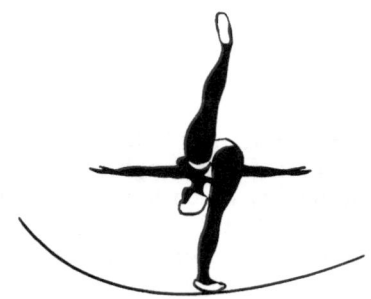

The balance of justice – even concerning women – can be very delicate.

Bibliography

Beumer, F. J. A. (1981). *Patient en Recht*. (Deventer, the Netherlands: Kluwer)
Declaration of Helsinki, Recommendation guiding medical doctors in biomedical research involving human subjects. Adopted by the 18th World Medical Assembly, Helsinki, Finland 1964, and as revised by the 29th World Medical Assembly, Tokyo, Japan, 1975

Declaration of the Medical Research Council. (1982). *Br. Med. J.,* **285**.

Human Rights and Scientific and Technological Developments, Report of the Secretary-General. Commission of human rights, 26th session, March 1970

Leenen, H. J. J. (1978). *Rechten van Mensen in de Gezondheidszorg.* pp. 82–102, (Alphen a/d Rijn, the Netherlands: Samson)

Leenen, H. J. J. (1981). *Gezondheidszorg en Recht.* pp. 124–38, 268–71. (Alphen a/d Rijn, the Netherlands: Samson)

Proceedings of the Boerhaavecursus 'Medische experimenten op Mensen', Leiden, January 1983

15
Psychosocial aspects of VIP in historical perspective: a case study of North-East Scotland

B. THOMPSON, R. ILLSLEY and R. HALLIWELL

INTRODUCTION

Aberdeen, a coastal city in North-East Scotland, has significance in relation to abortion in the United Kingdom (UK) for three reasons. First, a policy of abortion and sterilization was gradually introduced in the 30 years preceding the passing of abortion legislation in 1967. Secondly, records of nearly all pregnancy events have been maintained since 1951 for the whole community. Thirdly, a wide range of research projects relating to abortion, and attitudes concerned with the process of making decisions, and the experiences of both professionals and consumers have been undertaken over the years by obstetricians, psychiatrists and sociologists separately and in collaboration.

In recent years international data on the legal status of abortion and statistics for different countries have become available in world reviews of induced abortion (Tietze, 1981). Whatever the law, however, practise depends on how the situation is interpreted. The very uneven availability of abortion within the National Health Service (NHS) in the UK was highlighted by the 'Report of the Committee on the Working of the Abortion Act' (HMSO, 1974). Aberdeen became known for its liberal policy on abortion and sterilization starting in the late 1930s with the pioneer effort of Sir Dugald Baird, Professor of Obstetrics and Gynecology from 1938 to 1965, and continued by his successor, Professor Ian MacGillivray (Baird, 1965, 1971, 1975). Before the Abortion Act 1967 came into force in May 1968, the abortion policy in Aberdeen was carried out under the Common Law of Scotland. In order to establish that they acted 'in good faith' the gynecologists routinely involved the psychiatrists. Few consultants elsewhere in Scotland availed themselves of this freedom given by the difference between English and Scottish law.

A major interdisciplinary study was undertaken in Aberdeen when the debate on proposed legislation was in full swing. More gynecologists throughout Britain were moving cautiously towards a selective policy of termination, although discussion was guarded and information sparse

(Horobin, 1973). The study found that abortion commonly resulted in sociopsychological benefit, but that regrets and distress frequently followed when abortion was refused. It is rare for the type of experience and documentation found in Aberdeen on voluntary interruption of pregnancy (VIP) to be available prior to specific legislation. Hence its importance when the Abortion Act was being formulated (Simms and Hindell, 1971) and attempts to restrict the law debated (Marsh and Chambers, 1981). However, dramatic changes have occurred in abortion in Aberdeen in the 30 years between 1951 and 1980, and these are illustrated in this paper.

THE BACKGROUND

Aberdeen is a well-defined urban centre for administration, commerce and education with an extensive rural hinterland and is predominantly Protestant. In the 30 years under review the population has ranged from 200 000 to 220 000 and has become diversified as a result of the development of North Sea oil industry but, even now, about two-thirds of maternity patients have been born and raised in the city. The medical services are centralized and the total maternity services are co-ordinated. Only a few abortions, which occur in the one private general nursing home, are excluded from the records of pregnancy events occurring in the city involving local residents. Occasionally, for personal reasons, such as anonymity, a woman may prefer to leave Aberdeen to have an abortion. She may request that her doctor or the gynecologist refer her elsewhere or go elsewhere independently. The compilation of the Aberdeen Maternity and Neo-Natal Data Bank (Samphier and Thompson, 1981) indicates that there is little attempt to conceal VIPs irrespective of where they were performed.

RESULTS

All pregnancies

Pregnancy outcomes between 1951 and 1980 in five 6-year periods reveal the proportion of VIPs increased from 2 % to 19 % (Table 15.1) and the numbers from 426 to 3651. The rise started before the liberal Abortion Act came into force. After the Act the proportion of VIPs rose, paralleled by a decline in births. The proportion of 'other abortions' has remained fairly constant, with a slight increase in the late 1960s. These will not be discussed further but it is worth noting that septic abortions were seldom seen in the 1970s.

During the 30 years the characteristics of the women having a VIP have shown two opposing trends. *First*, a marked decrease occurred in three characteristics (Figure 15.1). The majority of VIPs in the 1950s were carried out in conjunction with sterilization. Most of the women were over 30 years of age and had several children. These married women, often severely debilitated, were offered termination and sterilization by obstetricians subject to concurrence by the psychiatrists. Most were the wives of semi-skilled or unskilled

Table 15.1 Percentage pregnancy outcomes (births, VIPs, other abortions) from 1951 to 1980 in 6-year periods

Period (6 years)	Pregnancy outcomes			
	VIP	Birth	Other abortions	All pregnancies Number (100%)
1951–56	2	91	7	22417
1957–62	2	91	7	23247
1963–68[1]	3	88	9	23081
1669–74	13	79	8	21708
1975–80	19	74	7	18873

[1] Abortion Act 1967 came into force May 1968

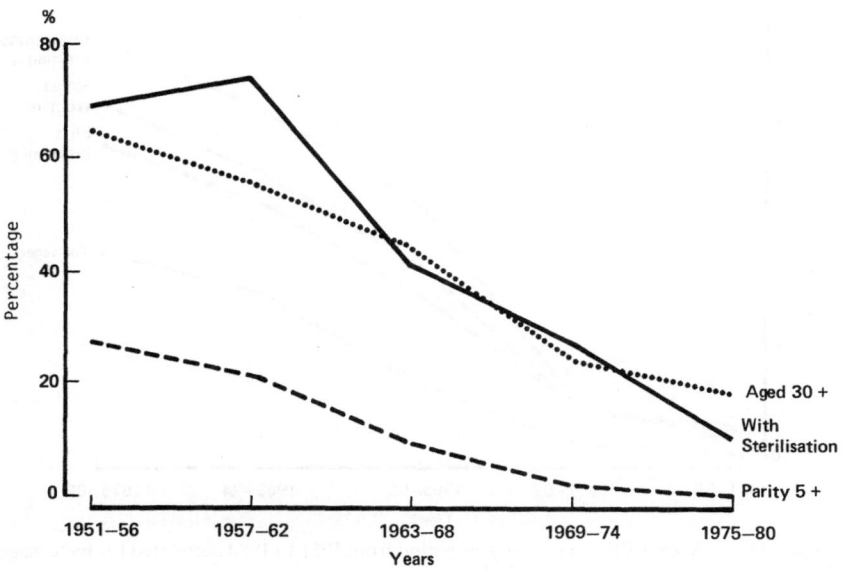

Figure 15.1 Percentage VIPs in each 6-year period from 1951 to 1980 by age, with concurrent sterilization and parity 5+

(other) manual workers (Table 15.2). Women in the upper social groups would have been offended if sterilization had been suggested (Thompson and Illsley, 1959). In the early 1950s, 7 out of 1000 pregnancies to wives of non-manual workers ended in VIP as compared to 21 out of 1000 pregnancies to wives of semi-skilled and unskilled manual workers. The ratio has increased in all groups but the differential between occupational groups has almost disappeared at a time when a two- or three-child family is the norm in Aberdeen (Pritchard and Thompson, 1982).

Table 15.2 Ratio of VIPs per 1000 pregnancies[1] for married women within husbands' occupational groups

	Husbands' occupational group		
Period	Non-manual	Skilled manual	Other manual
1951–56	7	11	21
1957–62	9	14	29
1963–68	17	23	27
1969–74	42	62	79
1970–80	56	63	63

[1] Births plus VIPs

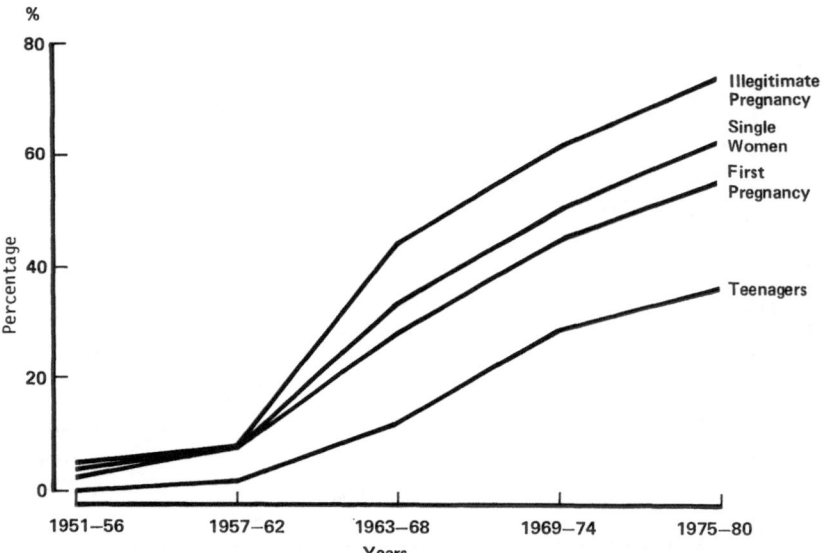

Figure 15.2 Percent VIPs in each 6-year period from 1951 to 1980 accounted for by teenagers, first pregnancies, single women and illegitimate pregnancies

Table 15.3 Rates of VIPs per 1000 women aged between 15 and 44, and 15 and 19, in census years 1951, 1961, 1966, 1971, 1980[1]

Census year	VIPs per 1000 women aged 15–44	VIPs per 1000 women aged 15–19
1951	2.0	—
1961	1.5	—
1966	2.8	2.4
1971	9.4	9.9
1980[1]	15.9	26.3

[1] Based on Census 1981 preliminary data

Four characteristics showed a marked increase – illegitimate pregnancies, most of which were to single women, in first pregnancies and women aged under 20, i.e. teenagers (Figure 15.2). Rates of VIP in women aged 15–44, and in teenagers, can be calculated for five census years from 1951 (Table 15.3). The rise in the late 1970s was particularly dramatic among teenagers (26.3 in 1980 compared to 15.9 for all women aged 15–44).

First pregnancies to single women

Most pregnancies to single women are first pregnancies. Single women, assuming that they do not abort spontaneously, have three possible outcomes – either marry and legitimate the baby, have an illegitimate baby, or have the pregnancy terminated. In the 1970s VIP increasingly offset the decrease in marriage during pregnancy without greatly affecting the proportion ending in an illegitimate birth (Pritchard and Thompson, 1982), By 1980 over half of first pregnancies to single women ended in abortion (Table 15.4).

There are, however, marked differences in behavior between occupational groups (Thompson, 1977; Illsley, 1980). If the first pregnancies to single women are divided according to the woman's occupational group, 80 % of those to women in professional occupations and students are now terminated (Figure 15.3). This applies to only 30 % of those to semi-skilled or unskilled manual workers, a similar proportion to that among professional women and students over a decade ago.

These figures reflect not only different behavior in the occupational groups in requesting abortion, but also the greater understanding and sympathy of doctors towards women from their own social milieu (Aitken-Swan, 1977). The outcome of pregnancy is the end-point of a chain of social action and social and medical decision-making (Horobin and Thompson, 1977). A crucial influence in the process is the 'moral characters' attributed to the women (Macintyre, 1977). The lower occupational groups, particularly those working in the traditional fishing industry among whom it was statistically deviant to marry before becoming pregnant (Thompson, 1956), came only slowly to request and obtain an abortion. The case for abortion from the different social groups was differently presented and differently perceived by those ultimately responsible for the decision (Aitken-Swan, 1973, 1977).

Table 15.4 Percentage of births – legitimate and illegitimate – and VIPs for first pregnancies to women single at conception in each 6-year period from 1963 to 1980

	First pregnancy outcomes			
	Birth			All first pregnancies
Period	Legitimate	Illegitimate	VIP	Number (100%)
1963–68	68	23	7	2860
1969–74	48	22	30	3799
1975–80	26	22	52	2891

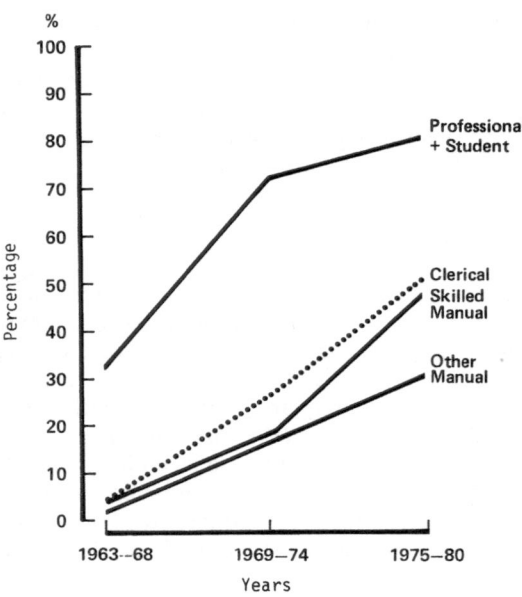

Figure 15.3 First pregnancies to women single at conception within occupational groups: percent age terminated

Making the decision

Once women themselves began taking the initiative in requesting VIP, the consultants found themselves in an ambiguous position. In the late 1960s, 37 % of women referred to them did not have a VIP performed. This fell to 10 % in 1980 and there is no doubt that over the years the accumulation of research findings from Aberdeen and elsewhere (see Illsley and Hall, 1976) has influenced the decisions made by the clinicians. Today VIP is seldom refused unless the pregnancy is 'too far advanced.' As single women, particularly manual workers, are more likely to request VIP later in pregnancy, this tends to perpetuate the differentiation against them. It is important to note that gynecologists vary in what they consider is 'too late.'

Nowadays about half the women who are referred for abortion, do not have it. They either cancel the initial appointment or do not appear for the scheduled operation. Increasingly women come 'too early' and are found to be not pregnant.

Contraception and VIP

There is little evidence that Aberdeen women rely on abortion instead of using contraception. Aberdeen has had a distinguished history in providing contraception for women since the 1920s and particularly since a local authority family planning clinic was opened in 1946. Only the diaphragm, unacceptable to most women, was available until oral contraception and the IUD were introduced in 1964 (Thompson, 1977). In 1974 the NHS accepted responsibility for providing contraception. The clinic was taken over and general practitioners were formally involved in family planning. By 1980, over 90 % of maternity patients had some experience with 'the Pill.'

In the late 1970s, 12 % of VIPs were repeats, nearly all being second VIPs, and 90 % of the first ones had been performed in Aberdeen. Repeats included most of the 2 % of VIPs which followed failed sterilization or pregnancy occurring with an IUD *in situ.* There has always been a vigorous policy to ensure that women having a VIP were properly informed about contraception and given every encouragement to use the services (Aitken-Swan, 1977).

Influence of medical innovation

In recent years about 3 % of VIPs in Aberdeen have been performed for fetal anomalies following innovations in methods of detection.

Medical innovations have also changed the VIP procedures. In the 1950s, 60 % of VIPs involved a major abdominal operation and about 10 days in hospital. Most were hysterotomies performed in conjunction with tubal ligation and there were a few hysterectomies (Table 15.5). The remaining 40 % were done by D&C. By the 1980s these operations were superseded by suction (87 %) and saline/prostaglandin (12 %) procedures. Hysterotomy, 'outdated as a method of terminating pregnancy' (Nottage and Liston, 1975) was rarely performed.

Table 15.5 Percentage of each VIP procedure for each 6-year period between 1951 and 1980

	VIP procedure					
Period	Hysterotomy and sterilization	D&C	Other[1]	Saline/ prostaglandin	Suction	Total (%)
1951–56	53	40	7	—	—	100
1957–62	68	16	15	1	—	100
1963–68	40	22	7	23	8	100
1969–74	12	4	1	12	71	100
1975–80	—	—	1	12	87	100

[1] Hysterotomy alone, pregnant hysterectomy, etc.

Findings accumulated on the complications of adjustment to sterilization if performed in conjunction with VIP (Thompson and Baird, 1968). Also possible coercion to agree to sterilization as a condition of VIP was widely deplored (Peel and Potts, 1969). With the development of laparoscopic sterilization as a day procedure and increasingly in the 1970s the alternative of vasectomy (47 % of all sterilization in 1980) the two issues of VIP and sterilization became divorced. The category of 'termination and concurrent sterilization' has had to be abandoned from a prospective study of sterilization designed in the mid-1970s for lack of couples experiencing this.

CONCLUDING REMARKS

The experience with VIP in Aberdeen played an important part when legislation was being considered or reviewed. Although this historical aspect should not be underestimated, for practical purposes the early experiences are irrelevant today. In spite of its history, Aberdeen is no longer atypical in the abortion scene in UK, and is still far from achieving the objective of 'every pregnancy a wanted pregnancy.'

The meaning of VIP has changed in the 30 years. The scene has been transformed under the impact of abortion legislation; medical innovations; the introduction, greater accessibility, and choice of widely acceptable contraception; and the alternative between laparoscopic sterilization or vasectomy. The radical change in the characteristics of women having a VIP, from the extremes of older, high-parity, lower social class mother to the unmarried, upper social class teenager pregnant for the first time, demonstrates the cultural revolution in attitudes and practices in sexual behavior, marriage and family formation which has occurred throughout society since the early 1960s (Dunnell, 1979; Illsley and Taylor, 1975). The outcomes have depended on decisions taken by individual doctors on medical issues confused by social, moral and ethical considerations.

It is because of differing cultural, religious and legal rules, and the strength of their enforcement, that abortion has a different meaning not only from country to country but from place to place and from one period to another. Thus while overall comparison may be useful, accurate interpretation depends on knowledge of the total situation and an understanding of the complex behavior and processes involved.

References

Aitken-Swan, J. (1973). The woman's story: married women; single women. In Horobin, G. (ed.) *Experience with Abortion*. pp. 96–164. (Cambridge: Cambridge University Press)

Aitken-Swan, J. (1977). *Fertility Control and the Medical Profession*. (London: Croom Helm)

Baird, D. (1965). A fifth freedom? *Br. Med. J.*, **2**, 1141–8

Baird, D. (1971). The obstetrician and society. The Galton Lecture, 1970. *J. Biosoc. Sci.*, Suppl. 3, pp. 93–111

Baird, D. (1975). The changing pattern of human reproduction in Scotland, 1928–72. *J. Biosoc. Sci.*, **7**, 77–97

Dunnell, K. (1979). *Family Formation 1976*. (London: H. M. Stationery Office)

H. M. Stationery Office (1974). *Report of the Committee on the Working of the Abortion Act*. Cmnd. 5579, 3 volumes. (London: HMSO)

Horobin, G. (ed.) (1973). *Experience with Abortion: A Case Study in North East Scotland*. (Cambridge: Cambridge University Press)

Horobin, G. and Thompson, B. (1977). Clearing the termination hurdles in the NHS obstacle course. *Health Soc. Ser. J.*, 772–3

Illsley, R. (1980) *Professional or Public Health: Sociology in Health and Medicine*. (London: Nuffield Provincial Hospitals Trust)

Illsley, R. and Hall, M. H. (1976). Psychosocial aspects of abortion: a review of issues and needed research. *Bull. World Health Org.*, **53**, 83–106

Illsley, R. and Taylor, R. (1975). Sociological aspects of teenage pregnancy. Summarized in *Pregnancy and Abortion in Adolescence*, WHO Technical Series Report 583 (Geneva)

Macintyre, S. (1977). *Single and Pregnant*. (London: Croom Helm)

Marsh, D. and Chambers, J. (1981). *Abortion Politics*. (London: Junction Books)

Nottage, B. J. and Liston, W. A. (1975). A review of 700 hysterotomies. *Br. J. Obstet. Gynaecol.*, **82**, 310–13

Peel, J. and Potts, M. (1969). *Textbook of Contraceptive Practice*. (Cambridge: Cambridge University Press)

Pritchard, C. and Thompson, B. (1982). Starting a family in Aberdeen 1961–79: the significance of illegitimacy and abortion. *J. Biosoc. Sci.*, **14**, 127–39

Samphier, M. L. and Thompson, B. (1981). The Aberdeen Maternity and Neo-natal Data Bank. In Mednick, S. A. and Baert, A. E. (eds.) *Prospective Longitudinal Research*. pp. 60–5. (Oxford: Oxford University Press)

Simms, M. and Hindell, K. (1971). *Abortion Law Reformed*. (London: Peter Owen)

Thompson, B. (1956). Social study of illegitimate maternities. *Br. J. Prev. Soc. Med.*, **10**, 75–87

Thompson, B. (1977). Problems of abortion in Britain – Aberdeen, a case study. *Pop. Stud.*, **31**, 143–54

Thompson, B. and Baird, D. (1968). Follow-up of 186 sterilised women. *Lancet*, **1**, 1023–7

Thompson, B. and Illsley, R. (1969). Family growth in Aberdeen. *J. Biosoc. Sci.*, **1**, 23–9

Tietze, C. (1981). *Induced Abortion: A World Review 1981*. (New York: The Population Council)

16
Legal aspects of abortion

M. M. BAYLSON

Abortion is a medical procedure which has significant social and legal connotations. More than any other medical procedure, abortion raises significant questions concerning the origin of human life, and the degree of freedom a woman should have over the consequences of intercourse and conception. Abortion impacts on the social significance of fertility and the birth rate in a particular country. The role of the physician varies. Depending upon the laws in effect, the physician may be properly serving the health needs of a patient, or may be circumventing laws prohibiting abortion enacted by a particular country.

The physician's role in influencing the availability of abortion is crucial. Legislatures and courts rely heavily on medical publications and the scientific findings of medical experience in determining which abortions to allow and which to prohibit, but medical findings are not sufficient. Social, religious or moral values are also important. Some people find abortions analogous to the medical 'experiments' of the Nazis. Others view abortions as essential to save the physical and mental health of a woman. A physician may decide to remain 'neutral' about the relative social values and legal aspects of abortion, but only perform them as a medical procedure. A short introduction to the legal history of abortion regulation, and a comparison of the laws of different countries, will help focus on the current controversy.

The several alternative legal–social–medical relationships concerning abortion include: (1) abortion is solely a decision by a patient with her physician, as to which there are no legal consequences whatsoever; (2) the physician is acting under certain well-defined medical standards which determine whether or not an abortion would or could be performed; (3) the availability of abortion is determined by the legislature or courts, as a matter of social policy or legal rule for a particular country; and (4) abortion is not the subject of legislative action, but significant other religious or social mores are in operation that either facilitate or preclude a woman's ability to have an abortion.

REGULATION OF ABORTION

Abortion in ancient times

Classical Greece and Rome did not prohibit induced abortion. In fact it was practiced quite commonly for economic reasons, for shame at illegitimacy, for fear of childbirth ruining the beauty of the mother, and when pregnancy and childbirth might endanger the health of the mother. It was recommended by both Plato and Aristotle as a means to limit the population of a state beyond a certain optimum, the latter going so far as to suggest compulsory abortion for a woman who already had her allotted number of children. Nor did the Hebrews of Old Testament times have anything to say against (or about) abortion. The Hippocratic Oath, however, seems to have forbidden it.

In the early years of Christianity, abortions were not illegal as long as the fetus was not 'formed' or 'animated' (a date which has changed over the years as medical science advanced). It was not until the seventeenth century that the opinion was put forward that the rational soul must be infused in the first moment of conception, and that even therapeutic abortion began to be completely prohibited in Canon law.

Abortion at common law

In the earlier stages of the common law (the legal heritage which governs most English-speaking countries), there were no prohibitions against abortions, up until the stage of 'quickening' which was usually defined as 14 weeks after conception. After 14 weeks, abortion was a misdemeanor (a relatively minor crime) but the law was hardly ever enforced.

Several legislative restrictions on the availability of abortions were passed in England and other English-speaking countries in the nineteenth and early twentieth century. However, the actual common law legal practice was reflected by the instructions which the judge gave in a celebrated 1938 criminal case against Dr Bourne, an English obstetrician, who performed an abortion, knowing that it would attract attention and possibly criminal prosecution, because he believed that childbearing would make his patient a 'mental wreck.'

At the time, under a British law, abortions were illegal unless they were designed to save the 'life' of the mother. The judge instructed the jury that 'life' concerned not simply the fact of life, but also the quality of life, meaning physical and mental health. The judge told the jury it could consider, as legitimate, the physician's view that continued pregnancy would make the woman 'a physical or mental wreck.' In Bourne, the jury acquitted Dr Bourne and no appeal by the prosecution was allowed.

The Bourne rationale was followed in the United States, for example, in a 1944 case, *Commonwealth of Massachusetts* v. *Wheeler*, where the court assumed the legality of therapeutic abortions 'whenever a risk of injury to the physical or mental health of the pregnant woman is greater than if the pregnancy were terminating.'

The essence of the Bourne decision has been adopted in other decisions in common law countries, as it relates to the physician's subjective, bona fide belief that the physician was acting in the best interest of the mother. For example, in a prosecution against a physician performing an abortion one court charged the jury that 'the doctor is entitled to take into account the social circumstances of the patient, . . . together with all other relevant circumstances pertaining to the patient and arriving at a genuine opinion as to whether the continuation of the pregnancy proposes a threat to her health.'

Abortion in the USA

The status of abortion legislation in the USA is as follows:

Prior to 1850   No state legislation restricting abortion

By 1900   Every state has made abortions criminal

By 1973   Four states (N.Y., Washington, Alaska, Hawaii) have removed most restrictions on abortions. Thirteen states have legislation permitting abortion in some circumstances (see below)

1973   US Supreme Court opinion prohibiting states from preventing first trimester abortions.

The legislation enacted by 13 states, based on the American Law Institute's Model Penal Code, permitted abortions where:

(1) the pregnancy threatened the woman's life;
(2) it involved a substantial risk that its continuance would impair the physical or mental health of the mother;
(3) the child will be born physically or mentally defective; and
(4) the pregnancy resulted from rape or incest.

1983 – STATUS OF LEGAL REGULATIONS

The laws currently in effect in four nations are compared in Table 16.1:

Table 16.1 Comparison of selected current abortion laws

USA	United Kingdom	Germany	People's Republic of China
First trimester: no restrictions allowed; second trimester: state may regulate if reasonable for maternal health	Abortions forbidden since 1976 1967 unless special circumstances present (see below)	Abortions forbidden since 1976 unless special circumstances present (see below)	First trimester: abortions allowed since 1957 if mother has not had abortion in the previous year and mother will not suffer from abortion

149

United States

In the Supreme Court's 1973 opinion, entitled *Roe* v. *Wade*, the Court set out the current rules binding on all states regarding abortion. Critics of the decision attacked the Court's action because it was acting as a legislature enacting a statute. Indeed, there has always been significant criticism of the Supreme Court for 'legislating' rather than deciding specific disputes, which is the traditional function of a court of law. The Supreme Court's holding is definitive. During the first trimester the abortion decision and its effectuation must be left to the medical judgment of the pregnant woman's attending physician. No state regulation is allowed. Subsequent to the end of the first trimester, the State, in promoting its interest in the health of the mother, may, if it chooses, regulate the abortion procedure in ways that are reasonably related to maternal health. Thereafter, the State may regulate and even prohibit abortion except where it is necessary, in appropriate medical judgment, for the preservation of the life and health of the mother.

The constitutional origin of the *Roe* v. *Wade* opinion goes back to the decision of the United States Supreme Court in *Griswold* v. *Connecticut* in 1965 in which the Court, for the first time, enunciated a constitutionally-based 'right of privacy.' The Court held that 'privacy' was a 'fundamental right' which meant that an individual's 'privacy' was entitled to the highest degree of constitutional protection. Under United States constitutional law, attempts to interfere with 'fundamental rights' are subject to 'strict scrutiny' by a reviewing Court. Interference with such rights is unconstitutional unless there is no rational basis between the asserted right and the constitutional protection which it deserves.

The United States Supreme Court held the right of privacy as the constitutional source of a woman's right to have an abortion. The Supreme Court cited the possible medical harm, psychological harm, a distressful life, problems of an unwanted child, and in some cases the stigma of unwanted motherhood. 'All these are factors a woman and a physician will consider in consultation.'

The Supreme Court, in the abortion cases, also specifically held that the unborn fetus is not a 'person' within the protection guaranteed under the Fourteenth Amendment to the United States Constitution. The Supreme Court also held that it was not necessary to resolve the 'difficult question of when life begins.' However, the Court held that the State acquired a legitimate interest in protecting 'potential life' at the end of the second trimester when the fetus has become viable.

In the abortion cases decided by the Supreme Court in June 1983 (*City of Akron*), a majority of the Court strongly reaffirmed the absolute right of a woman to a first trimester abortion, and held a number of state regulations on second trimester abortions invalid as not medically necessary. Medical literature, particularly the Standards for Obstetric and Gynecological Sciences published by the American College of Obstetricians and Gynecologicists, was heavily relied upon by the Court.

Some minimal regulations are allowed in the first trimester if they have no significant impact on a woman's exercise of the right to an abortion, and are justified by important State health objectives. Two examples of valid first trimester requirements are a simple informed written consent and the physician keeping records.

During the second trimester the State may not require that an abortion be done only in a hospital, but may outlaw abortions done in a physician's private office. In 1983 the court noted that medical literature had shown second trimester abortions had become much safer than in 1973. Thus, ambulatory outpatient clinics are perfectly reasonable for maternal health, at least in the early weeks of the second trimester.

The Court held invalid a State requirement that a pregnant woman under the age of 15 must obtain the informed written consent of one of her parents or her legal guardian, because the State law did not recognize that some minors under age 15 may be mature enough to make the decision themselves. A requirement of an overly detailed informed consent procedure was held too restrictive and an improper intrusion upon the discretion of the pregnant woman's physician. Also held improper was a 24-hour waiting period between the signing of a consent form and performance of an abortion; and a requirement of 'humane and sanitary' disposal of the remains of an unborn child.

The recent case-by-case development in the United States of a constitutionally-based 'right of privacy' is an important example of the tremendous power of the United States Supreme Court. The legal aspects of this power need not be reviewed here, but the impact of this power on the relationship between a physician and a patient is readily apparent.

The Supreme Court has, by the 'constitutionalization' of the 'right of privacy,' thrown the cloak of constitutional protection over many personal affairs, including, along with abortion, other relationships between the patient and physician. For example, the right to have a particular medical procedure or operation, such as artificial insemination, sterilization, or a sex change operation, and perhaps even the termination of life when based upon a rational medical choice, is now arguably constitutionally protected from governmental interference.

British Commonwealth

The British Abortion Act of 1967 is generally considered to be a reform of prior law. Many other Commonwealth countries have similar laws. Abortions are forbidden unless they qualify because of the presence of one or more of the following:

(1) risk to the life and grave risk to the health of the woman (the strict necessity indication);
(2) risk to physical or mental health from continuation of pregnancy, meaning risk beyond that normally associated with pregnancy (the therapeutic indication);
(3) some degree of likely serious physical or mental impairment of a child if born (the fetal indication);

(4) pregnancy by rape or incest (the juridical indication);
(5) the effect of childbirth upon the health and welfare of the woman's existing children and family (the social, sociomedical or socioeconomic indication);
(6) jeopardy to the social position of the woman or her family (the family indication);
(7) failure of a routinely employed contraceptive means (the contraceptive indication).

In addition to the above, there are also legislative implementation regulations such as: (1) gestational limits; (2) the qualification and expansion of the practioners; (3) approval procedures (hospital boards, etc.); (4) facilities; (5) third party consents (parents or purported father); (6) conscientious objection by the physician (in Britain this is not allowed if there is a serious danger to health of the woman presented to a physician); (7) citizenship or residency; (8) reporting requirements and confidentiality.

West Germany

Under traditional German law an abortion for medical reasons, i.e. when necessary to perserve the life and health of the pregnant woman,was not illegal.

Abortion was debated in Germany during 1963 into the 1970s. In 1975 the West German Federal Constitutional Court ruled that a German statute allowing abortion was unconstitutional because it violated the constitutional rights of unborn children. This law allowed an abortion during the first 12 weeks after conception if performed by a licensed physician and with the consent of the pregnant woman. An abortion was permissible in between 12 and 24 weeks if warranted by medical or eugenic indications.

The German court, contrary to the United States Supreme Court, specifically held 'life in the sense of historical existence of a human individual exists according to definite biological–physiological knowledge in any case from the 14th day after conception.' Part of the reasoning of the German court was that the German statute did not affirm the dignity of an unborn life, and suggested that a formal statutory condemnation of abortion is necessary to foreclose any inference that destruction of fetal life during the first 12 weeks of pregnancy is morally or legally a permissible act.

The new German law of 1976 also allows, in addition to legal abortion for medical reasons relating to mother's life and health, without time limit, abortions for medical reasons related to physical and mental defects in the child (within 22 weeks) and ethical–criminal reasons such as rape (within 12 weeks). The new law also permits abortion for social reasons (i.e. if there exists for the mother the danger of any other special circumstances of distress within 12 weeks).

One of the important factors in the present German law is a 'refusal' clause under which parties, including physicians, may refuse to participate in the performance of an abortion.

The People's Republic of China

By 1957 the Ministry of Health had stipulated the conditions shown in Table 16.1 above for *rengong liuchan* ('induced slipping delivery'), or abortion.

Contraception counselling was required as part of the operation. Now, abortion seems to be available on demand by the woman alone, and advocated by the State as a means of population control. No legislation can be found on the subject.

CURRENT LEGAL ISSUES

The fact that laws on abortion vary greatly requires physicians to be alert and knowledgeable on these issues: (1) specific laws regulating abortions in a particular jurisdiction; (2) particular record-keeping requirements; (3) specificity of the patient's consent; (4) consent of others in addition to the patient; (5) availability and legality of third party payment; (6) ethical duty of physician to patient *vis à vis* legal restrictions; (7) economic conditions of the mother; (8) conditions which may allow or justify the physician's decision to perform an otherwise illegal abortion, such as rape, incest, life of mother in danger, physical and/or mental health of mother in danger; possibility of a deformed fetus.

CONCLUDING REMARKS

What is the significance of these legal restrictions on decision-making within the physician—patient relationship? Perhaps depending on one's views on the mortality or propriety of abortions, artificial insemination, sex change operations, etc. — many judicial decisions champion the rights of individuals to have the best available medical science treat them in the way that they and their physicians think best. Obviously, it would be wrong to put the physician in the position of a policeman, to regulate the patient's morals or sexual practices. Generally, in the common law countries the function of the legislature is to establish social and moral standards. The broad outlines of a constitution are designed to preserve individual rights and practices. In the United States, the Supreme Court serves as the final arbitrator as to whether legislation is unduly restrictive on the rights of individuals. The balancing test may be a precarious one, and is usually better done by a legislature than a Court. However, this principle does not require a Court which has the ultimate authority of upholding the laws and Constitution of a sovereign country, to abdicate its authority.

Bibliography

Dickens, B. M. and Cook, R. J. (1979). Development of Commonwealth abortion laws. *Int. Compar. Law Q.*, **28**, 424–57

Horton, K. C. (1979). Abortion law reform in the German Federal Republic. *Int. Compar. Law Q.*, **28**, 288–96.

Issacs, S. L. (1980–81). The law of fertility regulation in the United States: A 1980 review. *J. Fam. Law*, **19**, 65–96

Kommers, D. P. (1977). Abortion and constitution: United States and West Germany. *Am. J. Compar. Law*, **25**, 255–85

Luk, B. H. (1977). Abortion in Chinese Law. *Am. J. Compar. Law*, **25**, 372–92

Mathews, M. (1976). Quantitative interference with the right to life: abortion and Irish law. *Catholic Lawyer*, **22**, 344–58

Robertson, J. A. (1983). Procreative liberty and the control of Conception pregnancy and childbirth. *69 Virginia L. R.*, 405–64.

Robbins, J. (1973). Unmet needs in family planning: a world survey. *Fam. Plann. Perspect.*, **5**, 232

World Health Organization (1978). *Induced Abortion*. WHO Technical Report Series 632, p. 5

17
Law and Abortion in Italy

M. FILICORI, C. FLAMIGNI and E. SAVIOTTI

In May of 1978 the Parliament of Italy approved a new abortion legislation that permits to obtain first trimester abortion on request. The law went into effect at the beginning of June 1978; in 1979, the first year of its full application, 187 400 legal abortions were performed (Filicori and Flamigni, 1981). Several political groups with different, sometimes opposing, political orientation soon began campaigning for changing parts of the abortion law, or for its total repeal. In an unprecedented political situation, both the Radical Party and the 'Pro-life' movement eventually proposed three different referenda to be submitted to the vote of the Italian people. If approved, the proposals from the 'Pro-life' movement would have severely restricted or totally eliminated the availability of legal abortion; the Radical Party proposal would have resulted in a more subtle but critical change: possibly it would have made legalized abortion more easily available, but much of the social implications of the law would be lost. In order to clarify the scope of each referendum and to understand the issues involved, it is necessary to examine in detail the Italian abortion law.

THE LAW NO. 194 OF 22 MAY 1978

The Italian abortion law contains 22 articles that can be essentially divided into four parts:

(1) an introduction where the basic principles of the law are enunciated;
(2) a series of specific guidelines which indicate the administrative steps to be followed in the application of the law, the cases that are subjected to specific regulations (e.g. minors, mentally retarded), the health facilities allowed to carry out legal abortions, and the procedures for requesting the status of conscientious objector;
(3) directions for the reporting of the epidemiological data resulting from the application of the law, and instructions for the creation of educational programs for health professionals; and
(4) a list of penalties for the abortion procedures accomplished in violation of the law.

155

The law is founded on the principle that the act of reproduction is a conscious and responsible choice; however, pregnancy termination should not be considered as a birth control method. The public family planning clinics (created in 1975) are requested to play an important role in the implementation of the law, as the primary source of information, counseling and support for the pregnant woman in relation to the economic and social provisions available. If possible, the clinic should intervene to help the woman to overcome the conditions determining the abortion request. The last paragraph of Article 2 specifically indicates that contraceptives can be prescribed to minors (below 18 years of age). The second part of the law (Articles 4–10 and 12–14) deals with its specific implementation. The principal divide set by the law is according to the length of pregnancy: below 90 days an abortion can be requested for a wide range of health, socioeconomic, judicial, or eugenic reasons. Moreover, in the first trimester an abortion can be obtained regardless of the grounds of the request after 7 days from the initial physician's consultation. Therefore, in this gestational period legal abortion is practically avaiable on request. It is interesting to notice that the law does not specify whether the gestational age should be calculated in days from the last menstrual period (LMP) or from the presumed day of conception. Furthermore, 90 days is almost 13 weeks, and not the limit of 12 weeks usually assigned to the first trimester. As a result, with an extensive interpretation of the law legal abortion may be obtained on request up to the 15th week of pregnancy. A large number of second trimester abortions are performed in the 12th–15th week, worldwide (Tietze, 1981); if in Italy many abortions at this gestational age are classified as 'within 90 days,' this might account for the apparent very low incidence of second trimester abortions (Filicori and Flamigni, 1981). Such attitude would be a consequence of the limited grounds for obtaining an abortion in the second trimester: life-threatening conditions related to the pregnancy, or medically proven fetal malformations or anomalies. The above conditions must be documented by an obstetrician–gynecologist. If an immediate threat to the woman's life exists, such documentation can be omitted. The problem of minors requesting an abortion is specifically dealt with in Article 12. For these women the consent of the parent or guardian is required by law. However, in a case where the parents deny such permission, or when the direct parent consultation is deemed unfeasible, the abortion procedure can be authorized by the juvenile judge. Urgent procedures exempt the woman from obtaining either the parental or the judicial consent. If the minor is in the second trimester of pregnancy the limits set for this gestational age also apply.

A similar procedure applies in the case of mentally retarded women. The husband, the guardian, or the woman herself can request the voluntary abortion by applying to the local court. In the case that the request is not submitted by the woman herself, she still must assent to the procedure. Like in the instance of minors, the judge must decide within 5 days.

As stated in Article 10, all diagnostic and therapeutic procedures involved and related to voluntary pregnancy termination are covered by the National Health Service and the Regional Administrations. Health facilities authorized to carry out legal abortions include public family planning clinics (the

Consultori Familiari), public hospitals, and private hospitals specifically licensed by the Regional Administrations.

Under the penalty of law (jail terms up to 3 years), voluntary abortion is forbidden outside the above-mentioned facilities. Therefore, unlike other countries, in Italy there has been no legal involvement of private physicians in induced abortion, and it is believed by some political groups (e.g. the Radical Party) that this has been a major factor contributing to the uneven implementation of the law in Italy.

The health personnel (physicians and nurses) of the facilities that offer abortion services can choose not to participate in the abortion procedures if this is against their moral principles. They can register as conscientious objectors by informing the local health authority and the hospital's director of their decision. However, conscientious objection cannot be invoked if emergency life-threatening conditions exist, and is limited to the abortion diagnostic and therapeutic procedures; pre- and post-abortion assistance and care cannot be denied on this basis; the status of objector is automatically void by the participation in routine abortion procedures; higher sentences are imposed for illegal abortions done by registered conscientious objectors.

Articles 11 and 16 deal with the official reporting procedures. The health facilities must transmit the statistical data (with names omitted) regarding each pregnancy termination to the local health authority. The Regional Administrations collect this information and relay it to the Ministry of Health within the month of January of each year. Thereafter, within February, the Minister of Health is required to present to the Parliament a report on the application of the abortion law. Most regions are not capable of providing statistical data within this rigorous deadline and, as a result, complete information is available only 13–16 months after the completion of the calendar year.

The problem of the adequate training of health personnel is critical when new medical procedures are suddenly introduced, as in the case of induced abortion. The Regional Administrations are invited to collaborate with the universities and the hospitals to organize educational programs in the field of human reproduction (Article 15). The first of these courses was held at the University of Bologna in September 1980 (Flamigni and Filicori, 1981).

Finally, Articles 17–22 list the penalties and terms for abortions not carried out according to the pesent law, and therefore illegal.

THE RESTRICTIVE PROPOSITION

Since its introduction in 1978, integralist Catholic groups campaigned to repeal or limit the extent of the abortion law. On the other side of the political arena, the Radical Party in 1980 began collecting signatures for a different referendum proposition calling for more accessible legal abortions. This delicate issue was made even more complicated by the fact that the 'Pro-life' movement had called for two separate referenda: the so-called 'maximal' and 'minimal' propositions.

The 'maximal' proposition

In 1975 the Supreme Court of Italy had ruled that when a woman is exposed to serious health threats in relation to her pregnancy, voluntary abortion is permissible. If approved, the changes of the 'maximal' proposition would have turned back the Italian abortion legislation to the pre-1975 conditions: illegal voluntary abortion with no exceptions. However, in Italy a referendum proposal cannot deal with Constitutional amendments, nor can it rule against the principles indicated by the Constitution. As this proposal did not take into consideration the 1975 Supreme Court ruling that the right to health of a pregnant woman overrides that of an unborn fetus, it would have been *de facto* anti-Constitutional. For this reason, the maximal proposition was never submitted to the Italian people, although it received far more than the 500 000 signatures needed for requesting a referendum.

The 'minimal' proposition

This proposition, which took into consideration the 1975 Supreme Court decision, would have limited legal abortion to those cases in which the life or the physical (not psychological) health of the pregnant woman is endangered. Abortion would have been forbidden on any other ground. No distinctions were made regarding the age of the woman, the duration of pregnancy, or mental retardation. No provisions existed for fetal malformation, or circumstances such as rape or incest. Voluntary abortion would have been punished with jail terms of up to 3 years; the woman undergoing an illegal abortion could receive a $100 fine. It is interesting to note that among the articles to be deleted by this proposition were those dealing with the upgrading of the health professional's training, not only in the field of abortion techniques but also of contraception and family planning.

THE DEREGULATING PROPOSITION

Despite the rapid increase in the incidence of legal voluntary abortion several difficulties and limitations appeared soon after the introduction of the 1978 law. Because of the high recourse to conscientious objection, and the uneven distribution of health facilities, it became clear that it was difficult to obtain an abortion in most southern regions. Even in those areas of the north with adequate abortion services it could take days, if not weeks, from the initial application to the abortion procedure. The limitation that abortion can be obtained only in public facilities and the lack of an economic incentive was blamed by the Radical Party for such delays. Their proposition would have cancelled all mentions of the type of facilities where abortion can be obtained and the administrative procedures to be followed. Therefore physicians would have been free to charge for abortions, though the procedures carried out in public facilities would still be covered by regional funds. As before, second trimester abortions would be allowed only in cases of serious threats for the pregnant woman or for fetal malformations, but the requirement for a detailed medical documentation would disappear. Regulations on minors and mentally handicapped would also be cancelled by the deregulating proposition. Paradoxically, this would have resulted in more difficulties for minors who requested an abortion, because of the abolished clause that the juvenile judge can overrule the parent's decision and has to decide on the matter within 5 days. The requirement of a consent signed by the parent or guardian for a surgical procedure such as abortion would still be binding. A referendum can only abrogate a law or parts of it, with no addition to the existing legislation; the Radical Party was planning on proposing new specific and more liberal regulations on minors, had the referendum been approved. Finally, all references to the epidemiologic reporting system would have been cancelled, as well as the formal requirement to provide family planning counselling to the woman seeking an abortion.

The political movement (in which the Radical Party itself had participated) that supported the 1978 abortion law put great emphasis on the social implications of induced abortion. One of the most relevant principles of the Italian law is the support offered to all pregnant women, whether or not they decide to bring to term their pregnancy. The community is therefore required to offer the best social and health protections to fulfill the Constitutional principle that all citizens have a right to health. From these premises stem the provisions that abortion must be free of charge and entrusted to public facilities. Public family planning clinics are called to play an ever-increasing role in the prevention and the management of voluntary abortion. The deregulating proposition would have deprived the abortion law of much of its social content. Moreover, by relieving public facilities from social pressures, this legislative change would probably have curtailed the number of public abortion services just in those parts of the nation where the need is greatest, with no assurance that private facilities would take over. As a result, the gap in the availability of safe abortion services between the north and the south of Italy could have worsened.

THE APPLICATION OF THE ABORTION LAW AND THE RESULTS OF THE REFERENDUM

Since the introduction of the new law in 1978, a high number of Italian women resorted to legal abortion (Filicori and Flamigni, 1981) despite the scarcity of public facilities specifically devoted to this procedure. The abortion law went into effect only 2 weeks after its approval by the Parliament, and only a limited number of public hospitals provided this service since June 1978. However, 68 700 legal abortions were reported in 1978 and this number jumped to 187 400 in 1979 (Table 17.1).

After some initial hesitation the Catholic Church and hierarchy strongly participated in the campaign for the repeal of the Italian abortion law. Italy is a largely Catholic country and the influence of the Church, though decreasing, is still very strong. The complexity of the moral issue of abortion, and the possible confusion created by the two opposing referenda, led to a belief that the restrictive proposition could be approved. On the other hand it was

Table 17.1 Abortion statistics, Italy, 1978–79

	1978[1]		1979		
	Abortions	Abortion[2] ratio	Abortions	Abortion[2] ratio	Abortion[3] rate
Total	68 700	142	187 400	215	13.7
Northern Italy	39 000	201	97 600	283	15.7
Central Italy	14 900	172	41 300	265	15.8
Southern Italy	14 800	73	48 500	131	10.0

[1] June to December
[2] Ratio of abortions per 1000 abortions plus livebirths
[3] Ratio of abortions per 1000 women aged 15–49

apparent that the Radical Party proposal stood few chances. The referendum was held on 17 May 1981, and a large majority of the Italian population (79.6%) went to the polls. The results of the 1981 vote are shown in Table 17.2. As in the past, the participation in the polls was lower in the south than in the center and the north. Nevertheless, both propositions were defeated by 67.9% and 88.5% majorities respectively; only minor regional differences showed in the final results. The traditionally more conservative political attitudes of the south did not seem to affect the vote on abortion. These results are even more impressive and indicative, considering the higher occurrence of conscientious objections and apparently lower incidence of voluntary abortion in the southern regions.

The results of the vote indicate that the large majority of the Italian people wish to maintain the option of voluntary abortion. Also, the Italian voters proved able to draw the subtle line that divides an unrestricted legislation from a law that privileges an equitable social protection of all citizens.

Preliminary data (Ministry of Health, 1981) show that 112 350 legal abortions were carried out in the first semester of 1980 in Italy. If the trend shown in the regions that already presented complete data for 1980 is maintained, a total number of about 220 000 legal abortions can be projected for 1980. This would raise the 1980 national abortion ratio (per 1000 known pregnancies) to 251, from 215 the previous year.

Table 17.2 Results of the abortion referendum, Italy, 17 May 1981

	Voters (percentage of total population of age)	Restrictive proposition (percentage against)	Deregulating proposition (percentage against)
Total	79.6	67.9	88.5
Northern Italy	86.4	67.1	88.9
Central Italy	85.0	72.8	90.1
Southern Italy (excluding Sicilia and Sardegna)	67.2	65.6	86.5
Sicilia and Sardegna	67.6	66.2	86.8

Acknowledgments

Dr Marco Filicori is the recipient of a Fulbright—Hays research grant, and of a travel grant from the Council for International Exchange of Scholars.

References

Filicori, M. and Flamigni, C. (1981). Legal abortion in Italy, 1978—1979. *Fam. Plann. Perspect.*, **12,** 228—31

Flamigni, C. and Filicori, M. (1981). *L'interruzione volontaria della Gravidanza.* (Palermo: Cofese)

Ministry of Health (1981). *Relazione al Parlamento sull'Applicazione della legge 22/5/1978, nr. 194; anno 1980.* Rome, 21 April

Tietze, C. (1981). *Induced Abortion; a World Review, 1981.* (New York: The Population Council)

18
Epilogue

E. S. E. HAFEZ

EPIDEMIOLOGICAL PARAMETERS

Extensive epidemiological studies have been conducted by the Population Council, Ford Foundation, Rockefeller Foundation and the Center for Disease Control (CDC) to evaluate the social and medical interactions of natality, fertility, family planning, morbidity, mortality and voluntary interruption of pregnancy (VIP). The 'epidemiologic transition theory' (Omran, 1982) describes four models of mortality and natality transition:

(1) the 'Classical Model' in the West where gradual declines in mortality (in the eighteenth and nineteenth centuries) was followed, after a lag of 50–75 years, by fertility declines which were also gradual; abortion played a small role in this model;
(2) the 'Accelerated Model' in Japan and eastern Europe where the lag was somewhat shortened and where fertility decline was significantly enhanced with widescale use of abortion;
(3) the 'Delayed Model' in the developing countries where mortality decline was delayed to the twentieth century while fertility continued at a high level: abortion prevalence in this model is relatively low;
(4) the 'Transitional Version' of the Delayed Model where fertility started to decline in recent decades in response to organized family planning efforts (with varying degrees of social development).

In 1965 family planning in western Europe was hardly accepted and the birth rate was relatively high. Ten years later family planning had become fully accepted and the birth rate had dropped by 35%. This rapid transition was due to several factors: an open atmosphere in sexuality; acceptance by family doctors, including services for teenagers; inclusion of family planning services in the National Health Insurance programs and fear that induced abortion might become the accepted family planning method (Kettings, 1982).

In developing countries abortions continue to be the major cause of mortality and morbidity in the childbearing age. Restrictive abortion laws force healthy women seeking an abortion to resort to life-threatening measures to terminate pregnancy. Procedures, even when done by physicians, are performed in unsterile conditions because of secrecy and the fear of heavy fines and the loss of license should they be discovered. Perforations by sharp instruments, chemical introduction into the systemic circulation, and renal and hepatic toxicity were the sequelae of these procedures (Rubin *et al.*, 1982). Hemorrhage, peritonitis and septicemia are frequent following any of the invasive techniques. Permanent sterility and chronic pelvic inflammatory disease is frequent in those patients who do not succumb.

PATTERNS OF INDUCED ABORTION

Rapid urbanization, the liberalization of customs, promiscuity in schools and universities, the lack of sex education and information about methods of contraception, the unavailability of family planning services and the absence of laws which favor the legalization of abortion are the chief causes of this increase. In countries where abortion is legal, maternal and child morbidity and mortality are only a quarter as high as in countries where abortion remains illegal; and if family planning services are available, morbidity and mortality are again reduced by half (Toumi, 1982). In the USA the number of abortion-related deaths has decreased dramatically since 1940, but sepsis has persisted. Unmarried adolescents who undergo incomplete abortion at 16 weeks gestation or more by intrauterine placement of a foreign body appear to have the highest risk of death from post-abortum infection (Grimes and Cates, 1982). Three of these risk factors (gestational age at the time of abortion, method, and completeness of abortion) can be influenced by medical personnel. Most Canadian women obtaining abortions are very young, unmarried and without previous deliveries. Many women obtain abortions early in gestation, which may be one of the reasons for the decline in abortion complications. The legalization of abortion did not seem to affect the age of first coitus and did not decrease the use of contraception during planned or unplanned coitus. The legalization of abortion did not appear to affect the ratio of pregnant women choosing to abort relative to those choosing to deliver, and did not decrease the incidence of illegitimacy (Diamond, 1982).

In certain Catholic and Moslem countries the highest percentages of induced abortions are recorded for women 31–35 years old with low education, and in women with medium income. In certain countries abortion is regarded and practiced as a form of contraception. The practice of folklore, rhythm and barrier methods are common, and the failure rate of these methods is high.

Government involvement to enact appropriate legislation to reduce pregnancy wastage, maternal morbidity and mortality is urged. This should include the provision of comprehensive family planning services, sex education and safe abortion services.

METHODOLOGY

Extensive investigations have been conducted on the application of prostaglandins, using different methods of administration, for voluntary termination of pregnancy (Amy, 1979, 1982; Amy et al., 1973; van den Bergh and Niermeijer, 1979; Karim, 1979; Karim and Amy, 1975, 1978; Kerenyi and Den, 1979; Schmidt-Gollwitzer et al.,1979). The relative potency, mode of application and side effects of various prostaglandin analogs are summarized in Tables 18.1 and 18.2. A combination of intracervical and extra-amniotic applied prostaglandin is an efficient method for treatment of intrauterine fetal death. Pretreatment of the cervix reduces the number of extra-amniotic applications necessary, minimizing the risk of an intrauterine infection. In contrast to systemic PG application, side effects due to local PG treatment are reduced.

The intra-amniotic instillation of a prostaglandin should not be regarded as the ultimate technique of mid-trimester abortion (Amy, 1982; Amy et al., 1982). It: (1) requires expertise; (2) cannot be used in patients with (a) ruptured membranes, (b) fetal death of more than 48–72 h duration, (c) hydatidiform mole; (3) effects strong uterine stimulation, but little ripening of the cervis; (4) causes a higher risk of excessive uterine bleeding after fetal expulsion.

It is likely that systemic administration of one of the more selective analogs (e.g. Sulprostone) is to be preferred.

The extra-amniotic ethacridine (Rivanol[R]; Farbwerke Hoechst AG Frankfurt, West Germany) –catheter method for mid-trimester abortion was first developed in Japan. Ethacridine (6,9-diamino-2-oxyetyl acridine lactate) is a yellow dye with antiseptic properties. 30–150 ml of a 0.1–0.2 % solution was used in combination with the insertion of a rubber catheter into the uterus. This method is effective in mid-trimester abortion and has been used extensively in Japan for many years without any serious complications (Ingemanson, 1982). The application of hysteroscopy was restricted by the need for general anesthesia, particularly to the pre- or post-abortum period, because the hyperemic atonic uterus is over-inflated, since monitoring with intrauterine pressure of only 5–10 mmHg. The indications for immediate post-abortum hysteroscopy are: (1) bleeding of unknown origin; (2) diagnoses of uterine septum or submucous fibroids in case of considering an immediate post-abortum IUD insertion, and (3) fractured forceps or suction cannula (van Lith et al., 1982). Post-abortum hysteroscopy should be performed under local anesthesia and intracervical epinephrine application.

Due to increased cost and morbidity from general anesthesia, local anesthesia provides an efficient, safe, and, in most cases, clinically satisfactory method of anesthesia for suction D&C. However, general anesthesia should continue to be considered in patients likely to be dissatisfied with local anesthesia.

The in vitro inhibitory effect of danazol, trilostane, azastene, cyanoketone, and WIN 32729 was tested on human placental enzymes. In vivo, danazol, administered to female volunteers prior to therapeutic abortion, caused decrease in serum progesterone, estradiol and DHAS levels (Rabe et al., 1982).

Abortifacients in primitive societies and in animal models

Acceptable abortifacients should have no effect on the mother but produce changes in the fetus. Primitive societies and tribes (Siway, Congo, Menomini,

Table 18.1 Characteristics and applications of major prostaglandins

Name	Major uses	Common routes	Manufacturer and Brand Names	Where registered
PGF$_{2\alpha}$	Second trimester abortion Labor induction To stop post-partum bleeding	IA, IV, EA IV IY	Upjohn 'Prostin F2 Alpha' ONO 'Prostarmon-F' ONO 'Prostaglan'	25 countries worldwide, including Australia, Brazil, Mexico, United Kingdom, USA Japan, Korea, Taiwan Brazil
15-Methyl-PGF$_{2\alpha}$ (tromethamine salt)	First and second trimester abortion Intrauterine death and mole *To stop post-partum bleeding*	IA, IM, VL, EA IM *IM*	Upjohn 'Prostin/15M'	India, USA
15-Methyl-PGF$_{2\alpha}$ methyl ester	*First and second trimester abortion* *Cervical dilatation before first trimester abortion*	*S, D* *S*	Upjohn	
PGE$_2$	Second trimester abortion Intrauterine death and mole Labor induction *Cervical dilatation before labor induction*	S, IA S, EA OT, VT *EA, OT, VT, EG, VG*	Upjohn 'Prostin E2' ONO 'Prostarmon-E' Upjohn UK 'Prostin E2' (OT)	15 countries worldwide (Europe, Western Hemisphere Pacific), including Guatemala, Hong Kong, UK, USA Japan, Korea, Taiwan UK

166

Compound	Uses	Routes	Company
16,16-Dimethyl-PGE$_2$	*First trimester abortion* *Cervical dilatation before first trimester abortion*	*S* *S, IM*	Upjohn Canada
16-Phenoxy-ω-tetranor-PGE$_2$ methyl sulfonyl-amide[2] (Sulprostone)	*First and second trimester abortion* *Cervical dilatation before first trimester abortion*	*IV, IM, EA* *IM, IC*	Schering AG
16, 16-Dimethyltrans-Δ2-PGE$_1$ methyl ester (ONO-802)	*First and second trimester abortion*	*S, EA*	ONO
9-Deoxo-16, 16-dimethyl-9-methylene-PGE$_2$	*First and second trimester abortion* *Cervical dilatation before first trimester abortion*	*S*	Upjohn

Uses and routes approved by at least one national drug regulatory agency appear in roman type; experimental uses, in italic type.
EA = extra-amniotic; IA = intra-amniotic; IM = intramuscular; IV = intravenous; S = vaginal suppository; D = vaginal device; OT = oral tablet; VT = oral tablet administered vaginally; VL = vaginal liquid; IC = intracervical; EG = endocervical gel; IY = intramyometrial; VG = vaginal gel.

Adapted from *Population Reports* Series G, No. 8; Population Information Program, The Johns Hopkins University, Baltimore, Maryland 21205, USA

Table 18.2 Deaths associated with abortion by intra-amniotic administration of a prostaglandin

Compound	Pre-existing conditions	Cause of death
$PGF^1_{2\alpha}$	Chronic alcoholism, pancreatitis; pontine myelolysis	Hematemesis + aspiration
$PGF^1_{2\alpha}$	Severe congestive heart failure	? Amniotic fluid embolism
$PGF^1_{2\alpha}$	Chronic hypertension; severe superimposed pre-eclampsia	Hypertensive crisis + cerebral hemorrhage
$PGF^1_{2\alpha}$	—	Intravenous narcotic + phenothiazine; respiratory arrest
Intravenous oxytocin + intra-amniotic Nacl + intra-amniotic $PGF^1_{2\alpha}$	—	Septicemia; DIC; acute tubular necrosis
$PGF^3_{2\alpha} + NaCl^2$	—	Septicemia; hemolysis or DIC
$PGF^3_{2\alpha}$	Grand multiparity	Uterine rupture; shock, death during hysterectomy
15-Methyl-$PGF^3_{2\alpha}$	Grand multiparity	Delayed post-abortal bleeding (day 12); shock; death during hysterectomy

[1] Cates *et al.*, 1977
[2] Adachi *et al.*, 1977
[3] Tejuja *et al.*, 1978

Jivaro, Masai, Baholol and Taulipany) utilized a variety of oral abortifacients: camel sputum, chopped hair of deer, ground toncadira ants in water, raw eggs, goat dung, amber and amber water, emetic of copper sulfate, iron sulfate solution (Devereaux, 1955). Inner bark of roots, juices of leaves, extracts, dried tubers and fruit of identified plants were also used as human oral abortifacients; parsley, klipsweet, caragute thistle, *Cabera manglias, Hibiscus* species, sigshi husca vine, *Acanthus* species, *Amplediacea cissus, Ephedra vulgaris, Casuarina equisetifolia* and *Cyperus kyllingia*. Various substances have been taken orally to produce self-induced abortion in women: abluent, aloes, ammonia, apiol, Beecham's pills, beer, camphor drops, caster oil, ergot of rye, gin, lavender, mustard opium tablets, penny royal pills, quinine, rosemary, stout, tanny tea and turpentine (Gebhard *et al.*, 1958). Several abortifacients have been used in experimental animals: actinomycin D, antigonadotrophin serum, antihistamines, antimetabolites, cadmium, cytotoxic agents, antimitotics; tissue poisons; ergot alkaloids, androgens, corticoids, estrogens, oxytocins, prostaglandins, sympatholytic agents, monoamine oxidase inhibitors and serotonins (Bennet, 1974).

There are remarkable species differences in the pharmacological responses of the myometrium during pregnancy suggesting special differences in two factors: (1) relative sensitivity of myometrium to progesterone block; and (2)

relative importance of ovaries and placentas in progesterone production at different stages of pregnancy. These difficulties should be evaluated when considering results on induction of abortion in various animal species and their relevance to man. The use of non-human primates, as in the animal model, may improve the predictability of animal toxicology and teratology. Inherent risks of chemical abortifacients include maternal ovarian genetic damage and fetal malformations, especially with antimitotic or antimetabolic drugs. The risks of serious maternal toxicity and side effects are high with most known abortifacients because of the difficulty in titrating a suitable therapeutic dose ratio among individual women.

CHROMOSOMAL ANOMALIES AND GENETIC COUNSELING

Nature often performs a sorting-out of fetuses with severe abnormalities by causing the mothers to spontaneously abort these pregnancies. However, some 1 million babies are born each year in the USA with diseases caused by genetic disorders (3 % of all births). Prenatal diagnosis is extensively used to detect several diseases: Down's syndrome, sickle-cell anemia (a blood disorder affecting blacks, causing death by age 45 for those who survive adolescence), spina bifida, and Tay-Sachs affecting one of 27 persons of European Jewish ancestry, appearing at 6 months and fatal to offspring within 4 years. Amniocentesis is performed between 14 and 18 weeks of pregnancy to test for genetic disorders. The percentages of 'false negative' and 'false positive' diagnoses are still unknown. In view of the increasing sophistication and accuracy of testing used for genetic counseling, several bioethical issues have arisen; for example, under what conditions should a fetus be aborted? Application of current knowledge and technology has increased capabilities for counseling and prenatal detection of various birth defects. The relative risk of occurrence of neural tube defects is summarized in Table 18.3.

The American College of Obstetrics/Gynecology (ACOG, 1982) has summarized the clinical significance as follows: embryonic and fetal serum contain a high concentration of AFP, a glycoprotein with a molecular weight of approximately 70 000 daltons. Alpha-fetoprotein is synthesized sequentially in the embryonic fetal yolk sac, developing gastrointestinal tract and liver. In normal pregnancy small amounts of this protein are transported into

Table 18.3   Relative risks of occurrence of neural tube defects (NTD) in the USA

Circumstances	Risk (incidence per 1000 births)
No family history of NTD	1
Positive family history – maternal	10
Positive family history – paternal	5
One parent with NTD	30
One prior infant with NTD	20
Two prior infants with NTD	60

Data from *Prenatal detection of neural tube defects* (1982), ACOG Technical Bulletin, No. 67

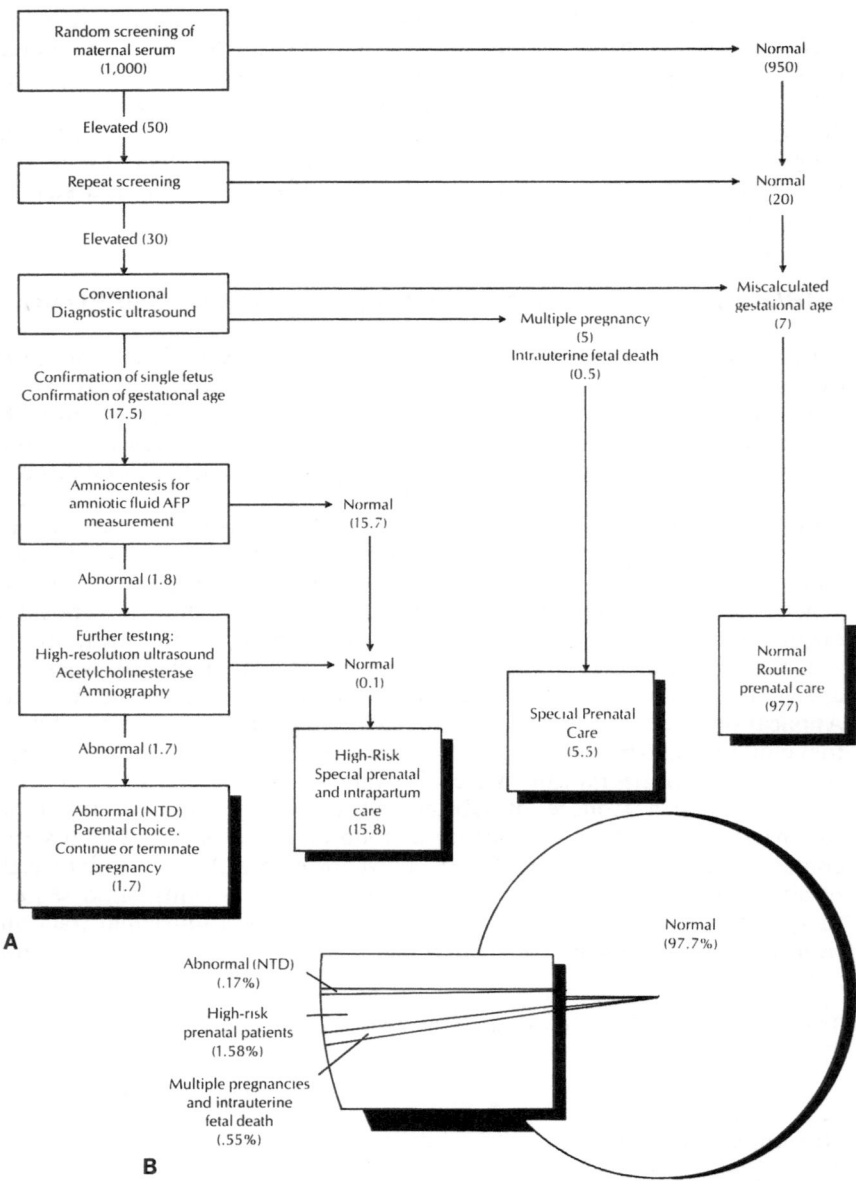

Fig. 18.1 Anticipated results of screening for neural tube defects in 1000 pregnant women (NTD prevalence, 1–2 per 1000). **A**: Screening procedure; **B**: screening results. Modified from Haddow, 1982 (with permission from Hospital Practice Publishing Company)

the amniotic fluid via fetal urination, gastrointestinal secretions, and transudation from exposed blood vessels. Alpha-fetoprotein is transported across the placenta causing low levels in maternal serum. The relative concentrations and general trends in the levels of AFP in fetal serum, amniotic fluid and maternal serum are of clinical significance during mid-gestation (15–24 weeks). The fetal serum concentration is highest at 15 weeks gestation and slowly declines during late pregnancy. Maternal serum AFP is low early in pregnancy but rises, reaching maximal levels at about 30 weeks gestation. Maternal serum AFP screening should be implemented only when it can be performed within a co-ordinated system of care which provides prompt, accurate diagnoses and appropriate follow-through services (Fig. 18.1). When such co-ordination of resources and services is not available the risks and cost appear to outweigh the advantages and the program should not be implemented (ACOG, 1982).

References

ACOG (1982). *Prenatal Detection of Neural Tube Defects*, Tech. Bull. 67

Adachi, A., Wilson, L. and Herzig, N. (1977). Prostaglandin $F_{2\alpha}$, hypertonic saline and oxytocin in midtrimester abortion. *N. Y. State J. Med.*, **77,** 46

Amy, J. J. (1979). Interruption de grossesse provoquee par les prostaglandines. In Amy, J. J. (ed.) *Les Prostaglandines et la Reproduction Humaine.* pp. 141–73. (Paris: Flammarion Medecine-Sciences)

Amy, J. J. (1982). Termination of second trimester pregnancy with prostaglandin analogues. In Keirse, M. J. N. C., Bennebroek, J., Gravenhorst, van Lith, D. A. F. and Embrey, M. P. (eds.) *Second Trimester Pregnancy Termination.* (The Hague: Leyde University Press/Martinus Nijhoff) (In press)

Amy, J. J., Karim, S. M. M. and Sivasamboo, R. (1973). Intra-amniotic administration of prostaglandin 15(S),15-methyl-E_2 methyl ester for termination of pregnancy. *J. Obstet. Gynaecol. Br. Commonw.*, **80,** 1017

Bennet, J. P. (1974). *Chemical Contraception.* (New York: Columbia University Press)

Cates, W., Jr., Grimes, D. A., Haber, R. J. and Tyler, C. W., Jr. (1977). Abortion deaths associated with the use of prostaglandin $F_{2\alpha}$. *Am. J. Obstet. Gynecol.*, **127,** 219–31

Devereaux, G. (1955). *A Study of Abortion in Primitive Societies.* p. 37. (New York: Julian)

Diamond, M. (1982). Abortion legalization and sexual and reproductive behavior. *Contracept. Deliv. Syst.*, **3** (3/4), Abstr. 430

Gebhard, P., Pomeroy, W., Martin, C. and Christenson, C. (1958). *Pregnancy, Birth and Abortion.* (New York: Harper & Row)

Grimes, D. A. and Cates, W., Jr. (1982). Fatal septic abortion in the United States (1975–1977). *Contracept. Deliv. Syst.*, **3** (3/4), Abstr. 429

Haddow, J. E. (1982). Screening for spinal defects. *Hosp. Prac.*, **17,** 128–38

Ingemanson, C. A. (1982). The ethacridine–catheter technique in second-trimester abortion. *Contracept. Deliv. Syst.*, **3** (3/4), Abstr. 451

Karim, S. M. M. (1979). Termination of second trimester pregnancy with prostaglandins, In Karim, S. M. M. (ed.) *Advances in Prostaglandin Research – Practical Applications of Prostaglandins and their Synthesis Inhibitors.* pp. 375–409. (Lancaster: MTP Press)

Karim, S. M. M. and Amy, J. J. (1975). Interruption of pregnancy with prostaglandins. In Karim, S. M. M. (ed.) *Advances in Prostaglandin Research – Prostaglandins and Reproduction.* pp. 77–148. (Lancaster: MTP Press)

Karim, S. M. M. and Amy, J. J. (1978). Prostaglandins and human reproduction. In MacDonald, R. R. (ed.) *Scientific Basis of Obstetrics and Gynaecology.* 2nd edn., pp. 345–92. (Edinburgh: Churchill Livingstone)

Kerenyi, T. D. and Den, T. (1979). Intraamniotic instillation of saline and prostaglandin for midtrimester abortion. In Zatuchni, G. I., Sciarra, J. J. and Speidel, J. J. (eds.) *Pregnancy*

Termination – Procedures, Safety, and New Developments. pp. 254–60. (Hagerstown: Harper & Row)

Kettings, E. (1982). Abortion and contraception in the Netherlands. *Contracept. Deliv. Syst.,* 3 (3/4), Abstr. 427

Omran, A. R. (1982). Health and population dynamics: the vital connection. *Contracept. Deliv. Syst.,* 3 (3/4), Abstr. 3

Population Reports (1982). Series G, No. 8, *Population Information Program.* Johns Hopkins University, Baltimore, MD 21205, USA

Rabe, T., Kiesel, L. and Runnebaum, B. (1982). *In vivo* and *in vitro* inhibition of placental progesterone synthesis by steroidogenic inhibitors. *Contracept. Deliv. Syst.,* 3 (3/4), Abstr. 445A

Rubin, A., Mbere, J. and Barrow, V. (1982). Abortion in South Africa. *Contracept. Deliv. Syst.,* 3 (3/4), Abstr. 415

Tejuja, S., Choudhury, S. D. and Manchanda, P. K. (1978). Use of intra- and extra-amniotic prostaglandins for the termination of pregnancies – reports of multicentric trial in India. *Contraception,* **18,** 641–52

Toumi, L. (1982). Complications of illegal abortion in Africa. *Contracept. Deliv. Syst.,* 3 (3/4), Abstr. 436

van den Bergh, A. S. and Niermeijer, O. (1979). Termination of advanced second trimester pregnancy with intraamniotic sulprostone, In Friebel, K., Schneider, H. and Wurfel, H. (eds.) *International Sulprostone Symposium.* pp. 119–20 (Berlin: Schering AG)

van Lith, D. A. F., van Schie, K. J., Beekhuizen, W., van der Pas, H. and Lindemann, H. J. (1982). Post second trimester abortion CO_2 hysteroscopy under local anesthesia. *Contracept. Deliv. Syst.,* 3 (3/4), Abstr. 439

Index

173